64.00

369 0240366

# The Hastings Center Guidelines for Decisions on Life-Sustaining Treatment and Care Near the End of Life

# The Hastings Center Guidelines for Decisions on Life-Sustaining Treatment and Care Near the End of Life

REVISED AND EXPANDED SECOND EDITION

BY

Nancy Berlinger, Bruce Jennings,
Susan M. Wolf

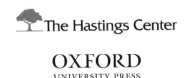 The Hastings Center

OXFORD
UNIVERSITY PRESS

# OXFORD
### UNIVERSITY PRESS

Oxford University Press is a department of the University of Oxford.
It furthers the University's objective of excellence in research, scholarship,
and education by publishing worldwide.

Oxford   New York
Auckland   Cape Town   Dar es Salaam   Hong Kong   Karachi
Kuala Lumpur   Madrid   Melbourne   Mexico City   Nairobi
New Delhi   Shanghai   Taipei   Toronto

With offices in
Argentina   Austria   Brazil   Chile   Czech Republic   France   Greece
Guatemala   Hungary   Italy   Japan   Poland   Portugal   Singapore
South Korea   Switzerland   Thailand   Turkey   Ukraine   Vietnam

Oxford is a registered trademark of Oxford University Press in the UK and certain other
countries.

Published in the United States of America by
Oxford University Press
198 Madison Avenue, New York, NY 10016

Library of Congress Cataloging-in-Publication Data
Berlinger, Nancy.
The Hastings Center guidelines for decisions on life-sustaining treatment and care
near the end of life / Nancy Berlinger, Bruce Jennings, and
Susan M. Wolf. — Rev. and expanded 2nd ed.
p. ; cm.
Guidelines for decisions on life-sustaining treatment and care near the end of life
Rev. ed. of: Guidelines on the termination of life-sustaining treatment and
the care of the dying / by the Hastings Center. c1987.
Includes bibliographical references and index.
ISBN 978–0–19–997456–6 (cl. : alk. paper) — ISBN 978–0–19–997455–9 (pbk. : alk. paper) —
ISBN 978–0–19–997457–3 (e-book)
I. Jennings, Bruce, 1949–   II. Wolf, Susan M.   III. Hastings Center.   IV. Guidelines on the
termination of life-sustaining treatment and the care of the dying.   V. Title.   VI. Title: Guidelines
for decisions on life-sustaining treatment and care near the end of life.
[DNLM:   1. Life Support Care—standards.   2. Decision Making.   3. Life Support
Care—ethics.   4. Terminal Care—ethics.   5. Terminal Care—standards. WX 162]
LC Classification not assigned
179.7—dc23
2012029054

To the memory of Julia M. Boltin
*et in Arcadia ego*

N.B.


To the memory of Hugh and Marge Jennings

B.J.


To the memory of my parents

S.M.W.

# Disclaimer

This material is not intended to be, and should not be considered, a substitute for ethics consultation or medical, legal, or other professional advice on particular cases or for particular institutions. While this material is designed to offer accurate information with respect to the subject matter covered and to be current as of the time it was written, research and knowledge about medical and health issues is constantly evolving. The publisher, the authors, and The Hastings Center make no representations or warranties to readers, express or implied, as to the accuracy or completeness of this material. The publisher, the authors, and The Hastings Center do not accept, and expressly disclaim, any responsibility for any liability, loss, or risk that may be claimed or incurred as a consequence of the use and/or application of any of the contents of this material.

# Contents

# Preface to the Second Edition

In January 2007, The Hastings Center launched a project to revise and expand our ethics guidelines on end-of-life care, first published in 1987. These *Guidelines* are the product of that project.

The 1987 *Guidelines on the Termination of Life-Sustaining Treatment and the Care of the Dying* (The Hastings Center and Indiana University Press) were the single most influential publication in The Hastings Center's history. They anticipated the development of clinical practice guidelines and other professional guidance for health care professionals, were influential in health law and policy, and were cited in United States Supreme Court Justice Sandra Day O'Connor's concurring opinion in the *Cruzan* decision (1990), a landmark legal case on end-of-life decision-making.

The major goal of this project has been updating and expanding the 1987 *Guidelines* to reflect the subsequent twenty-five years of empirical research, clinical innovation, legal and policy developments, and evolution of professional consensus concerning the practices and systems that can support ethically sound treatment decision-making and the delivery of safe, effective, and compassionate care near the end of life. The revised *Guidelines* also offer guidance on pediatric decision-making, a topic that was not addressed in the original edition. They reflect the contemporary landscape of ethics in health care settings, including the institutional ethics services that patients, their surrogates and loved ones, and health care professionals should be able to use. These *Guidelines* also reflect continuing efforts over the past two and a half decades to organize health care around the interests of patients and in ways that respect patients' families and social relationships. While these *Guidelines* address many specific scenarios in care near the end of life, they continually reinforce the importance of care planning and care coordination; clear, consistent, and fair processes for decision-making by patients and surrogates; the full integration of palliative care into treatment; the psychological and social dimensions of care near the end of life; and the need for institutional structures to support good care at the bedside.

Guidelines alone do not improve health care, including care near the end of life. The 1987 *Guidelines* were supported by the publication of a companion *Casebook* edited by Cynthia B. Cohen and published by Indiana University Press and by a subsequent six-year education project (Decisions Near the End of Life) in health care settings around the country, in collaboration with the Education Development Center. That was a time of growing public awareness of end-of-life decision-making as the result of litigation, federal and state policy-making, increased research and education, and realities including the HIV/AIDS epidemic. However, as The Hastings Center concluded in a 2005 report commissioned by the Robert Wood Johnson Foundation, greater awareness of the ethical dimensions of end-of-life care has not consistently translated into improved care; we still have a long way to go.[1]

As these revised *Guidelines* are published, our country is confronting the challenges of health care reform, an aging population, increasing technological capacity to extend life, and serious cost implications. It is time for a fresh look at end-of-life care that fully integrates the insights of ethics and law, medicine and other health care professions; the experiences of patients and family caregivers; and patient advocacy.

Guidelines can help create a shared commitment to critical thinking about clinical practice, and can support behavior change aimed at clinical, institutional, and social innovation. Guidelines can also help in times of crisis and times of reflection. In keeping with this, we have structured this document for ease of reference during difficult clinical situations, as we did in the 1987 *Guidelines*. We clarify the specific skills and areas of knowledge that health care professionals need so they can support informed decision-making and good care near the end of life. These *Guidelines* also strive to support institutional systems that deliver ethically competent care, including informational technologies and organizational approaches that build effective cooperation among professionals and other staff caring for a patient. Responsibility for the care of a patient near the end of life often changes hands during the course of a patient's end-of-life experience. The members of a patient's care team may not be in the same place at the same time. All can nonetheless share a vision of what good care is, a commitment to putting this vision into practice, and the ability to do so.

The 1987 *Guidelines* were the product of a Hastings Center project funded by Shirley Katzenbach. Susan M. Wolf, JD, served as Project Director and principal author of the *Guidelines* and Bruce Jennings, MA, served as Associate Project Director and a crucial contributor. The 1987 *Guidelines* were the consensus product of an interdisciplinary working group.

The revised edition of the *Guidelines* is again the product of a Hastings Center project, this time funded by a distribution from The Albert Sussman Charitable Remainder Annuity Trust and a major grant from The Patrick and Catherine Weldon Donaghue Medical Research Foundation. Additional support was provided by the donors to The Anika Papanek Memorial Fund at The Hastings Center, in memory of Anika Papanek (2000–2010), and by unrestricted donations to The Hastings Center. Nancy Berlinger, PhD, MDiv, has served as Project Director, with Bruce Jennings and Susan Wolf as Associate Project Directors. The revised *Guidelines* were drafted by these three, with extensive input from members of an interdisciplinary working group. The revised *Guidelines* are again a consensus document representing agreement among the working group members identified below. Working group members contributed countless insights during our meetings and through comments on successive drafts of the manuscript.

Several working group members deserve special thanks for their individual as well as their collaborative efforts on behalf of this project. Alan Meisel, JD, Sandra H. Johnson, JD, LLM, and Charles P. Sabatino, JD, shared their expertise on developments in law, regulation, and public policy. Their comments and clarifications contributed to the Introduction, sections of Parts One and Two, and the Cited Legal Authorities.

J. Randall Curtis, MD, MPH, provided guidance concerning many aspects of physician-patient communication and clinician education. The model process for family conferences described in Part Three, Section 1, is adapted with permission from his published clinical research. He participated in initial drafting and subsequent revisions of two subsections of Part Three, Section 4, on clinical aspects of withdrawing life-sustaining treatments and on mechanical ventilation. Daniel Sulmasy, MD, PhD, FACP, and Nessa Coyle, ANP-BC, ACHPN, PhD, FAAN, participated in initial drafting and subsequent revisions of the Part Three, Section 4 subsection on palliative sedation. Joseph J. Fins, MD, FACP, participated in the initial drafting of the subsection of Part Three, Section 4, on brain injuries and neurological states, and Kristi Kirschner, MD, participated in further development of that material.

Susan Block, MD, Julia Connelly, MD, and Nessa Coyle, ANP-BC, ACHPN, PhD, FAAN, also made important contributions to the development of sections of Part Three, by identifying communication issues and clinician education priorities in different care settings. Linda Emanuel, MD, PhD, provided important early feedback to guide the development of the advance care planning guidelines in Part Two, Section 1. Alan Fleischman, MD, and Raymond Barfield, MD, PhD, made vital contributions to the pediatric guidelines in Part Two, Section 3. The guidelines for ethics services, in Part Two, Section 6, are adapted with permission from the published work of Nancy Neveloff Dubler, LLB, and her coauthors.

Many other individuals, including our additional correspondents and three anonymous reviewers for Oxford University Press, contributed expert insights to this project. We are especially grateful to those individuals who consulted with us on the perspectives of persons living with disabilities, who may have more experience than most in making decisions involving life-sustaining treatments and technologies. Scholars in disability studies also offered important critical perspectives on concepts such as "dignity" and "quality of life," and raised important questions about whether an individual's quality of life can be assessed by someone other than the person living that life. To elicit these perspectives, the *Guidelines* project, in collaboration with the Donnelley Family Disability Ethics Program (now the Donnelley Ethics Program) at the Rehabilitation Institute of Chicago, held a consultation in July 2007 with local and national representatives of disability communities. (See Contributors.) The goal of this consultation was to explore issues in care near the end of life that were of particular concern to members of disability communities and those living with disabilities, and to collaboratively identify insights that should be incorporated into these *Guidelines*. This consultation led to the drafting of a working paper by project staff. All consultation participants had opportunities to review and comment on this paper in draft, including the terms of its use as background material for the project. Part One, Section 4; Part Two, Section 2; and Part Three, Sections 2 and 4, of these *Guidelines* make the most extensive use of this working paper, in discussing the social contexts of health care and the importance of integrating the perspectives of persons who make long-term use of life-sustaining treatments and technologies into guidelines on life-sustaining treatments and technologies near the end of life. We are grateful to all participants in this consultation (including those who have chosen not to be identified by name in this document), to the staff of the Donnelley Ethics Program, and to Kristi Kirschner, MD, and Adrienne Asch, PhD, MS, of our working group, for their profound contributions to these *Guidelines*.

*Hastings Center Report* Managing Editor Joyce Griffin assisted the authors in editing the *Guidelines* manuscript. Research Assistant Polo Black Golde, and his successor, Colleen Farrell, were tireless in their dedication to this project throughout their tenures at The Hastings Center. The project owes them, and Administrative Assistant Vicki Peyton, special thanks. Current and former Research Assistants Alison Jost, Jacob Moses, and Cameron Waldman and Project Interns Kieran Docherty, MBChB, Melissa Kurtz, MSN, MA, Nan Sze Ling, JD, Priya Katari, and Michael Gallinari also contributed to this project. We are extremely grateful to all.

Nancy Berlinger, Project Director
Bruce Jennings, Associate Project Director
Susan M. Wolf, Associate Project Director

# Contributors

Members of The Hastings Center Project on *Guidelines for Decisions on Life-Sustaining Treatment and Care Near the End of Life*

These individuals are responsible for the *Guidelines* that follow. Institutional affiliations are provided for identification purposes only.

**Project Director:**

**Nancy Berlinger, PhD, MDiv**
Research Scholar
The Hastings Center
Lecturer
Yale University School of Nursing

**Associate Project Directors:**

**Bruce Jennings, MA**
Director of Bioethics
Center for Humans and Nature
Lecturer
Yale University School of Public Health

**Susan M. Wolf, JD**
McKnight Presidential Professor of Law,
    Medicine & Public Policy
Faegre Baker Daniels Professor of Law
Professor of Medicine
Faculty Member, Center for Bioethics
Founding Chair, Consortium on Law and
    Values in Health, Environment &
    the Life Sciences
University of Minnesota

**Working Group:**

**Adrienne Asch, PhD, MS**
Director, Center for Ethics at Yeshiva
    University
Professor of Epidemiology and Population
    Health
Professor of Family and Social Medicine
Albert Einstein College of Medicine
Edward and Robin Milstein Professor of
    Bioethics
Yeshiva University

**Raymond Barfield, MD, PhD**
Associate Professor of Pediatrics and
    Christian Philosophy
Director, Pediatric Palliative Care
    Program
Schools of Medicine, Divinity and
    Nursing
Duke University

**Susan Block, MD**
Chair, Department of Psychosocial
  Oncology and Palliative Care
Dana-Farber Cancer Institute and Brigham
  and Women's Hospital
Co-Director, HMS Center for Palliative
  Care
Professor of Psychiatry and Medicine
Harvard Medical School

**Robert A. Burt, JD**
Alexander M. Bickel Professor
Yale Law School

**Julia Connelly, MD**
Medical Director, Orange County Nursing
  Home
Professor Emerita of Internal Medicine
University of Virginia Medical School

**Nessa Coyle, ANP-BC, ACHPN, PhD,
  FAAN**
Ethics Consultant
Memorial Sloan-Kettering Cancer Center

**J. Randall Curtis, MD, MPH**
Professor of Medicine
Section Head, Pulmonary and Critical
  Care Medicine
Harborview Medical Center
University of Washington

**Nancy Neveloff Dubler, LLB**
Consultant in Ethics, New York City
  Health and Hospitals Corporation
Senior Associate
Montefiore-Einstein Center for Bioethics
Professor Emerita of Bioethics
Albert Einstein College of Medicine

**Linda Emanuel, MD, PhD**
Director, Buehler Center on Aging,
  Health and Society
Feinberg School of Medicine
Northwestern University
Principal Investigator
Education for Physicians in End-of-Life
  Care (EPEC) Project

**Betty R. Ferrell, RN, PhD, FAAN,
  FPCN**
Professor of Nursing Research and
  Education
City of Hope
Research Scientist and Principal
  Investigator
End of Life Nursing Education
  Consortium (ELNEC)

**Joseph J. Fins, MD, FACP**
E. Williams Davis, Jr., M.D. Professor of
  Medical Ethics
Professor of Medicine, Professor of Public
  Health, and Professor of Medicine in
  Psychiatry
Weill Cornell Medical College
Director of Medical Ethics and Attending
  Physician
New York Presbyterian Hospital-Weill
  Cornell Center

**George Fitchett, DMin, PhD**
Director of Research and Professor
Department of Religion, Health, and
  Human Values
Rush University Medical Center

**Alan Fleischman, MD**
Clinical Professor of Pediatrics
Clinical Professor of Epidemiology and
  Population Health
Albert Einstein College of Medicine

**Carlos Gomez, MD, PhD (d. 2010)**
Former Medical Director
District of Columbia Pediatric Palliative
    Care Collaboration

**Sandra H. Johnson, JD, LLM**
Professor Emerita of Law and Health Care
    Ethics
Center for Health Law Studies
Saint Louis University School of Law

**Kristi L. Kirschner, MD**
Clinical Professor, Medical Humanities
    and Bioethics and
    Physical Medicine and Rehabilitation
Feinberg School of Medicine
Northwestern University
Former Director, Donnelley Family
    Disability Ethics Program
Rehabilitation Institute of Chicago

**Alan Meisel, JD**
Professor of Law
Dickie, McCamey, and Chilcote Professor
    of Bioethics
Director, Center for Bioethics and Health
    Law
University of Pittsburgh

**Richard Payne, MD**
Professor of Medicine and Divinity
Duke University

**Gloria Ramsey, JD, RN, FAAN**
Associate Professor
Graduate School of Nursing
PhD Program Director, Community
    Research Engagement
Center for Health Disparities Research
    and Education
Uniformed Services University of the
    Health Sciences

**Charles P. Sabatino, JD**
Director, Commission on Law and Aging
American Bar Association

**Colleen Scanlon, RN, MS, JD**
Senior Vice President for Advocacy
Catholic Health Initiatives

**Mildred Z. Solomon, EdD**
President and CEO, The Hastings Center
Clinical Professor of Anaesthesia and
Director, Fellowship in Medical Ethics
Department of Global Health and Social
    Medicine
Harvard Medical School

**Daniel Sulmasy, MD, PhD, FACP**
Clinton-Kilbride Professor of Medicine
    and Medical Ethics
Department of Medicine and Divinity
    School
Associate Director, The MacLean Center
    for Clinical Medical Ethics
University of Chicago

**Project Staff:**

**Polo Black Golde**
**Colleen Farrell**
**Alison Jost**
**Jacob Moses**
**Cameron Waldman**
Research Assistants

**Vicki Peyton**
Administrative Assistant

**Additional Meeting Participants:**
The individuals in this category are not
    responsible for the *Guidelines* that
    follow but provided important informa-
    tion and perspectives through consul-
    tation with the authors and Working
    Group, in collaboration with the

Donnelley Ethics Program (formerly the Donnelley Family Disability Ethics Program) at the Rehabilitation Institute of Chicago. Institutional affiliations are provided for identification purposes only. Nine other individuals, including two who have died, are not listed by name, as it was not possible to determine definitively whether they wished to be so listed. The authors are profoundly grateful to these individuals and to those acknowledged by name here.

**Rebecca Brashler, LCSW**
Director, Global Patient Services
Donnelley Ethics Program
Rehabilitation Institute of Chicago

**Carmen Cicchetti**
Business Support Manager
Assistive Technology Manager
Donnelley Ethics Program
Rehabilitation Institute of Chicago

**Steven M. Eidelman, MBA, MSW**
H. Rodney Sharp Professor of Human
    Services Policy and Leadership
Department of Human Development
Family Studies Faculty Director
National Leadership Consortium on
    Developmental Disabilities
University of Delaware

**Carol J. Gill, PhD**
Associate Professor
Department of Disability and Human
    Development
University of Illinois at Chicago

**Marilyn Golden**
Senior Policy Analyst
Disability Rights Education and Defense
    Fund (DREDF)

**Elizabeth Gould, MSW, LCSW**
Director, State Programs
Alzheimer's Association

**Debjani Mukherjee, PhD**
Director, Donnelley Ethics Program
Rehabilitation Institute of Chicago
Assistant Director of Graduate Studies
Medical Humanities and Bioethics
Assistant Professor of Physical Medicine
    and Rehabilitation, and of Medical
    Humanities and Bioethics
Feinberg School of Medicine
Northwestern University

**Teresa A. Savage, PhD, RN**
Consultant, Donnelley Ethics Program
Rehabilitation Institute of Chicago

**Marjorie Shultz, JD, MAT**
Professor Emerita of Law
Boalt Hall School of Law
University of California at Berkeley

**Additional Correspondents:**
The individuals in this category are not
    responsible for the *Guidelines* that
    follow but provided important information and perspectives on specific topics
    through consultation with the authors.
Institutional affiliations are provided for
    identification purposes only.

**Leslie Adams, MSW**
Social Worker, TrinityKids Care,
    Providence TrinityCare Hospice
Consultant, Children's Hospice and
    Palliative Care Coalition
Co-Coordinator, Southern California
    Pediatric Palliative Care Network

**Mary Ann Baily, PhD**
Fellow, The Hastings Center

**Carol Bayley, PhD**
Vice President for Ethics and Justice
    Education
Dignity Health

**Jessica Berg, JD, MPH**
Professor of Law, Bioethics, Public Health
Associate Director, Law-Medicine Center
Case Western Reserve University

**James L. Bernat, MD**
Louis and Ruth Frank Professor of
    Neuroscience
Professor of Neurology and Medicine
Dartmouth-Hitchcock Medical Center

**Kathy Brandt, MS**
Senior Vice President, Office of Education
    and Engagement
National Hospice and Palliative Care
    Organization

**Lori Butterworth**
Co-founder, Children's Hospice and
    Palliative Care Coalition
Founder, Jacob's Heart Children's Cancer
    Association

**Lewis Cohen, MD**
Professor of Psychiatry
Director, Renal Palliative Care Initiative
Tufts University School of Medicine

**Devon Dabbs**
Executive Director and Co-founder
Children's Hospice and Palliative Care
    Coalition

**Kathleen Foley, MD**
Pain and Palliative Care Service
Society of Memorial Sloan-Kettering
    Cancer Center Chair
Memorial Sloan-Kettering Cancer Center

**Sarah E. Friebert, MD, FAAP**
Director of Palliative Care
Akron Children's Hospital

**Elizabeth Gould, MSW, LCSW**
Director, State Programs
Alzheimer's Association

**Joanne Hatchett, MSN, RN, FNP**
Woodland Healthcare
Dignity Health

**Timothy Kirk, PhD**
Assistant Professor of Philosophy
York College, City University of New York

**Melissa J. Kurtz, RN, MSN, MA**
Bioethics Consultant
Montefiore Medical Center

**Hannah I. Lipman, MD, MS**
Chief, Bioethics Consultation Service
Associate Director, Montefiore-Einstein
    Center for Bioethics
Associate Professor of Clinical Medicine
Divisions of Geriatrics and Cardiology
Montefiore Medical Center

**Galen Miller, PhD**
Executive Vice President
National Hospice and Palliative Care
    Organization

**Alvin H. Moss, MD, FACP**
Director, Center for Health Ethics and
    Law
Professor of Medicine
Robert C. Byrd Health Sciences Center
West Virginia University

**Shirley Otis-Green, MSW, ACSW,
    LCSW, OSW-C**
Senior Research Specialist, Division of
    Nursing Research and Education
City of Hope

**Judi Lund Person, MPH**

Vice President, Compliance and
  Regulatory Leadership
National Hospice and Palliative Care
  Organization

**Thomas J. Smith, MD, FACP**

Massey Endowed Professor of Palliative
  Care Research and Medicine
Massey Cancer Center
Virginia Commonwealth University

**Joan M. Teno, MD, MS**

Professor of Health Services, Policy, and
  Practice
Professor of Medicine
Associate Director, Center for
  Gerontological and Health Care
  Research
Alpert School of Medicine
Brown University

**Rev. John F. Tuohey, PhD**

Regional Director and Endowed Chair in
  Applied Health Care Ethics
Providence Center for Health Care Ethics
Providence Health Care

**Gay Walker, RN**

Administrator, TrinityKids Care,
  Providence TrinityCare Hospice
Consultant, Children's Hospice and
  Palliative Care Coalition
Co-Coordinator, Southern California
  Pediatric Palliative Care Network

**Funders:**

The project to produce these revised
*Guidelines* was funded by a distribution
from The Albert Sussman Charitable
Remainder Annuity Trust and a major
grant from The Patrick and Catherine
Weldon Donaghue Medical Research
Foundation. Additional support
was provided by the donors to The
Anika Papanek Memorial Fund at
The Hastings Center, in memory of
Anika Papanek (2000–2010), and by
unrestricted donations to The Hastings
Center. We are deeply grateful to all
funders for their support.

# How These *Guidelines* Are Organized

This document consists of an Introduction followed by three Parts:

The Introduction describes the function and sources of ethics guidelines, including the ethical and legal foundations for these *Guidelines*. Key distinctions appear in distinctive typeface with explanations in standard typeface.

Part One presents the framework and context for these *Guidelines*, including the goals of care near the end of life, skills-based ethics competencies for health care professionals, the organizational systems that support good end-of-life care, and social, economic, and legal contexts. Goals and competencies appear in distinctive typeface with explanations in standard typeface.

Part Two builds on this framework to present the guidelines that are the heart of this document. These include guidelines on advance care planning, treatment decisions for adults and children, care transitions, determination of death, and institutional policy. Guidelines appear in distinctive typeface with explanations in standard typeface.

Part Three supports the implementation of these *Guidelines* with additional material on communication in end-of-life care.

The *Guidelines* include a Glossary, a list of Cited Legal Authorities, a Selected Bibliography, and an Index.

# Introduction

Decisions about the use of life-sustaining treatment when a person is seriously ill and likely to be near the end of life have profound consequences for that person, for his or her family and other loved ones, and often for health care providers.[2] These decisions will, to some extent, determine the time and circumstances of the person's death. And these decisions will shape the person's experience of remaining life—where it is lived, with whom, and with what degree of comfort or suffering. These decisions also have an inevitable social dimension. They compel us, as a society, to examine our common ethical priorities concerning the relief of suffering, what it means to live and to die, the rights of individuals, and the ultimate goals of medicine. They confront us with issues of justice, equity, and the economic constraints on the use of health care resources. The social dimensions of treatment decision-making near the end of life also include the cultural values, whether associated with religion, ethnicity, profession, or other identities and affiliations, which may inform how professionals present treatment options and how patients and surrogates make decisions.

Ethical challenges arise when the ethically appropriate course of action or range of choices is unclear, or when there are competing ethical claims that may not be reconcilable. Discussions about whether to use or forgo life-sustaining treatment frequently raise ethical concerns for health care professionals. These discussions and the resulting decisions should be informed by ethical norms and legal rights and protections concerning the health and welfare of some of the most vulnerable members of society; by health care goals that follow from these norms, rights, and protections; and by analysis based on the history of careful thinking, publication, and policy on end-of-life care. Our society must be confident that the decision-making processes used in health care institutions and by individual health care professionals are ethically sound, as well as equitable in the claims they allow any individual to make on shared health care resources.

These *Guidelines* are written for physicians, nurses, and other clinicians who care for patients facing decisions about life-sustaining treatment and patients nearing the end of life. These *Guidelines* are also intended to be useful to those responsible for the education of these clinicians, professionals who make institutional policy on care near the end of life, and public policy-makers working to improve end-of-life care. Patients, loved ones, and surrogate decision-makers may also find the *Guidelines* helpful.

## The Function and Sources of These Ethics Guidelines

Ethics guidelines are different from clinical practice guidelines and from law, although they are related to both of these. Ethics guidelines for end-of-life care are grounded in the moral traditions of medicine and nursing and are consistent with the moral traditions of other health care professions such as clinical social work and clinical psychology. They reflect broad ethical, religious, and legal traditions of American society as well as decades of research, deliberation, and consensus-building among professionals, policy-makers, and patients and loved ones. Their claim to serious attention derives from the informed and reasoned positions they present and from the widely acknowledged standards of ethically responsible clinical practice on which they are based.

These *Guidelines* do not provide a formula or algorithm for making correct decisions. They are not "cookbook" ethics. They aim to guide reflection, judgment, and action in providing good care near the end of life and, in particular, to provide an ethical framework for making decisions under conditions that are challenging and sometimes psychologically distressing. They clarify the rights and responsibilities of each participant in the decision-making process. They can help ensure that these decisions are made with the appropriate deliberation, transparency, and fair process, as well as safeguards for vulnerable patients. These *Guidelines* can help protect patients against both undertreatment, such as failing to provide medically appropriate interventions desired by the patient, and overtreatment, in the form of interventions that are unwanted by the patient or are unduly burdensome to that patient.

In formulating these *Guidelines*, we have been attentive to the state of the law. However, these *Guidelines* do not constitute legal advice. Users of this document should determine how the law in their jurisdiction bears on these ethical recommendations. Although these *Guidelines* differ from law in their status and authority, they can help policy-makers, legislators, regulators, and judges identify where more explicit legal direction is needed and where existing law impedes ethical decision-making, either directly or by creating uncertainty. These *Guidelines* may also offer model formulations that can be translated into the language of statutes, regulations, and judicial rulings. However, not all ethics standards need to be or should be written into law.

Health care professionals in the United States worry about lawsuits and even about the possibility of criminal prosecution. Although the law serves a legitimate function in setting limits to behavior, it is a mistake to allow health care, which exists to care for the sick and to relieve suffering, to be driven primarily by liability concerns. Legal counsel to hospitals and other health care institutions, and legal advisors to individual health care providers, have a responsibility, as lawyers with expertise in health law, to help ensure that health care is driven by patient-centered goals and that health care professionals are not preoccupied by legal concerns. These *Guidelines* thus offer guidance to health lawyers and to health care risk managers concerning their role in institutional policy-making to support good care near the end of life.

## Legal and Ethical Consensus Informing These *Guidelines*: Rights, Protections, and Key Philosophical Distinctions

The right of patients to forgo life-sustaining treatment has been recognized by law in the United States starting in the mid-1970s. This right is reflected in landmark cases such as *Quinlan* (producing the first state supreme court decision on end-of-life decision-making, in 1976) and *Cruzan* (producing the first U.S. Supreme Court decision on this issue, in 1990), in a large number of legal cases decided since *Quinlan*, and in federal and state statutes. Federal and state law recognize and authorize the use of advance directives, such as durable powers of attorney for health care decision-making (also known as proxy directives) and treatment directives (such as living wills). These allow patients to state in advance what treatments they do or do not want under different clinical circumstances, and who should act as their surrogate decision-maker, if they lose decision-making capacity. As the legal rules have been clarified, a parallel ethical consensus has developed. A broad ethical and legal consensus on much of end-of-life care is now in place. These *Guidelines* have been developed based on this legal and ethical consensus, which is summarized below.

**Patients with decision-making capacity have a common law and constitutional right to refuse life-sustaining treatment.**

The landmark *Quinlan* and *Cruzan* decisions, and many others, have established that patients have a legal right to refuse life-sustaining medical treatment. This right has been recognized both in common law rulings by judges and rulings based on the federal and state constitutions, and is broadly reflected in federal and state statutory law. (See Cited Legal Authorities.)

**Patients who lack decision-making capacity have the same rights to refuse life-sustaining treatment as patients with decision-making capacity. The manner in which these rights are exercised is different, as a surrogate decision-maker must usually speak for them.**

The *Quinlan* and *Cruzan* decisions, and subsequent case law and statutes, have also established that patients who lack decision-making capacity retain the right to refuse life-sustaining medical treatment. This right must usually be exercised by a surrogate decision-maker. The surrogate should decide based on the patient's prior explicit treatment preferences or, if these are unknown, the patient's preferences inferred from the surrogate's knowledge of and experience with the patient. If the surrogate lacks adequate basis for inferring those preferences, then the surrogate should decide based on the patient's best interests. Constitutional law, statutes, and judicial decisions authorize the use of advance directives and recognize surrogate decision-makers and standards for surrogate decision-making.

**The right to refuse life-sustaining medical treatment does not depend on projected life expectancy, whether long or short. Patients have a basic right to be free of unwanted treatments.**

Decisions about forgoing life-sustaining treatment usually arise when death is the unavoidable or probable outcome of the patient's underlying medical condition. However, a patient does not need to be categorized as "terminally ill," "actively dying," or "imminently dying" for these decisions to be ethically justified. Individuals have a basic right to be free of unwanted treatment no matter what their prognosis.

**There is no ethical difference between withholding and withdrawing life-sustaining medical treatment.**

The basic right to be free of unwanted treatment does not depend on whether a treatment has already started. A patient's right to refuse unwanted life-sustaining medical treatment can be exercised by opting to refrain from starting a treatment (withholding), or by opting to stop a treatment after it has been started (withdrawing). To decide to "forgo" a treatment may thus mean either deciding not to start a treatment or deciding to stop a treatment. Withholding and withdrawing may be different clinical and psychological experiences. Some health care professionals may perceive these differences as ethically challenging. However, recognizing their legal and moral equivalence is crucial. Relieving suffering, preventing burdens from unwanted or ineffective treatment, and respecting patients' wishes and preferences or best interests may motivate decisions to withhold a treatment, withdraw a treatment, or both.

**No treatment or form of care is intrinsically "ordinary" or "extraordinary."**

The benefits and burdens of a treatment from the patient's perspective determine the appropriateness of the treatment, regardless of whether the treatment is complex and technologically sophisticated or simpler and more routine. The assessment of the benefits and burdens of medical treatment *to the patient* has sometimes been cast in terms of "ordinary" and "extraordinary." This contrast has been understood in different ways, including morally required versus morally optional interventions, standard versus nonstandard care, or simple versus complex treatment. This traditional distinction and language has often confused decision-making and is now less frequently used than in the past. To avoid confusion and prevent burdens to patients resulting from unclear communication, the language of "benefits" and "burdens" is preferable. Patients have rights to refuse treatment, whether that treatment is simple or complex. The decision should hinge not on the simplicity or complexity of the treatment, but on the benefits and burdens of the treatment from the patient's perspective.

Palliative care is integral to good health care.

The relief of suffering is integral to the role of physicians and nurses as healers and caregivers and to health care as an ethical enterprise. Efforts to cure or manage disease are also efforts to prevent or relieve suffering caused by disease. Patients may experience a failure to relieve their suffering as a harm. All patients deserve expert treatment of their pain and symptoms, and respect as whole persons and social beings during the experience of illness. This is accomplished through the integration of interdisciplinary palliative care (including palliative medicine, palliative nursing, and other palliative professions) into medical treatment and patient care. As with other treatments, the benefits and burdens of a palliative intervention from the patient's perspective determine the appropriateness of that intervention. The Bibliography includes selections from the extensive literature on palliative care, including empirical research on the benefits of the early integration of palliative care into the treatment plan.

It is ethically acceptable to provide medication sufficient to control a patient's pain and symptoms even in the rare circumstance in which this intervention may foreseeably hasten the patient's death.

It is rare that medication properly administered with the intent of relieving pain and symptoms will hasten a patient's death. Available evidence suggests that when opioids are properly administered to relieve symptoms such as dyspnea or cancer pain, the respiratory depression that may occur is unlikely to lead to respiratory failure.[3] Even when medication intended to relieve pain and symptoms does have the foreseeable risk of hastening death, it is ethical for health care providers to prescribe and to administer the pain-relieving medication, following the rule of "double effect." This rule distinguishes between practices intended to relieve a patient's pain that may have a secondary, unintended effect of hastening death, and practices that are actually intended to bring about a patient's death. According to the rule of double effect, an action with two possible effects—one good, one bad—is ethically acceptable if four conditions are satisfied:

1. The action itself (here, administering the medication) is not morally wrong.
2. The action is undertaken with the sole intention of bringing about the good effect (here, relieving pain or symptoms) even if the bad effect (here, hastening death) is foreseeable.
3. The action does not bring about the good effect by means of the bad effect (here, that pain relief is not accomplished by ending life).
4. The reason for undertaking an action with two possible effects is clear and urgent (here, that there is a clinical need to administer this medication, at this dose, at this time, in order to relieve pain or symptoms).

Thus, administering medication with a risk of hastening death is morally acceptable if the purpose of doing so is the relief of pain or symptoms, the medication and dose are therapeutically necessary, and, as with any treatment, the patient or surrogate consents to the risk. For selections from the literature on double effect, refer to the Bibliography.

## Forgoing life-sustaining treatment is ethically and legally distinct from suicide, from euthanasia, and from physician-assisted suicide.

A patient's or surrogate's decision to forgo life-sustaining treatment and allow death to occur is not the ethical or legal equivalent of suicide. When health professionals implement a patient's or surrogate's decision to forgo life-sustaining treatment, they are not performing actions that are equivalent to killing the patient (euthanasia) or assisting the patient to end his or her own life by suicide. Although this distinction has occasioned debate, the right to refuse treatment is long settled and well established. Physician-assisted suicide and euthanasia have been far more controversial. A handful of U.S. states allow certain forms of physician-assisted suicide. No state allows euthanasia.

Changes in law and policy in three states since the mid-1990s mean that the legal and social context for these *Guidelines* differs somewhat from the context of the 1987 *Guidelines*, which stated that "[O]ur society forbids assisting suicide or active euthanasia, even if the motive is compassionate." This is still true of euthanasia. The landscape has changed to some extent for assisted suicide.

In 1997, the U.S. Supreme Court issued rulings in two cases (*Vacco v. Quill* and *Washington v. Glucksberg*) in which the Court rejected arguments that assisted suicide was a right protected under the U.S. Constitution. However, neither ruling prohibited states from enacting their own laws to permit assisted suicide. In 1997, the state of Oregon enacted the Death with Dignity Act, which permits terminally ill state residents "to end their lives through the voluntary self-administration of lethal medications, expressly prescribed by a physician for that purpose," thereby permitting physicians to assist in this act under these specific conditions. In 2009, the state of Washington enacted a similar Death with Dignity Act, which permits state residents with a life expectancy of less than six months "to request lethal doses of medication from medical and osteopathic physicians." In 2010, a decision by the Supreme Court of Montana (*Baxter v. Montana*) concluded that a physician who assisted a patient to end his or her own life voluntarily would not be liable for prosecution under that state's homicide statute. The evolving legal situation in Montana is related to, but distinct from, the Oregon and Washington statutes. (For citations, see Cited Legal Authorities.)

The practice authorized by statute in Oregon and Washington is known by various terms, including "assisted suicide," "physician aid-in-dying," "physician-assisted death," and "physician-assisted suicide." When referring to this practice, the authors of these *Guidelines* have chosen to use the term "physician-assisted suicide" (PAS) because this term seems to most clearly describe the two key features of what is authorized in these statutes, namely: 1) self-administration of a lethal dose of medication (i.e., suicide), when the medication and dose are 2) prescribed by a physician.

Avoiding confusion between the help or aid that physicians provide in the care of all dying patients and a specific practice authorized in two states has been our primary aim in making this choice of language. In our references to PAS, we have further sought to avoid language that obscures the legal and practical distinction between physician-*assisted* suicide and physician-*administered* euthanasia, which is illegal in the United States. We are mindful that some clinicians, scholars, and policy-makers use different terms (or more than one term), and that some commentators have clear preferences among these terms while others do not. We are also mindful that the word "suicide" has specific moral connotations for many members of American society. We conclude that no term is perfect, some terms are less clear or less common than others, and careful definition is crucial to informed discussion.

Published data from Oregon and Washington suggest that reported cases of physician-assisted suicide under those states' law and protocols are uncommon. In Oregon, for example, the 71 reported deaths that occurred under the provisions of that state's Death with Dignity Act in 2011 represented 22.5 deaths per 10,000 total deaths.[4] It should be noted that Oregon and Washington analyze and tabulate only those cases of physician-assisted suicide that are reported to them as such by physicians, so there may be additional unreported cases.

Health care professionals who care for dying patients in states where PAS is legal may face special ethical challenges. Institutional policy in these states should clarify the rights of patients under state law. This policy should also clarify the rights and responsibilities of physicians, other health care professionals, and institutions with respect both to participation in physician-assisted suicide and to a refusal to participate. The statutes in Oregon and Washington have prompted the development of explicit policies for institutions. Clinician education should support professionals' ability to obtain accurate information about relevant policies in the institutions in which they practice.

Published 2011 data from Oregon and Washington also suggest that most PAS deaths that occur in each state involve patients who are enrolled in hospice.[5] Institutional policy in states where PAS is legal should therefore clarify the responsibilities of hospice workers and hospice programs concerning how to provide good care to a hospice patient who is considering physician-assisted suicide and who wishes to remain enrolled in hospice for the remainder of his or her life. Clinician education in these states should offer hospice workers opportunities to discuss and reflect on the ethical and organizational challenges they may face in providing care to patients who are considering PAS and who disclose this information to hospice caregivers.

Professionals in every state should have opportunities to learn about and reflect on the continuing debate over PAS within American medicine and American society. Clinician education should take special care to describe the Oregon and Washington statutes and policies accurately to ensure that clinicians understand what practices are (and are not) permitted in these states.

These *Guidelines* discuss patient-initiated inquiries about physician-assisted suicide or euthanasia in Part Two, Section 2 ("Making the Decision at Hand"). The guidelines and commentary on conscientious objection by professionals and institutions in Part Two, Section 2 ("Conflicts and Challenges Related to Treatment Decision-Making") and Part Two, Section 6 ("Guidelines on Conflict Resolution") are relevant to refusals to participate in physician-assisted suicide. The Bibliography includes a selection of recent literature offering a range of clinical, ethical, and legal perspectives on physician-assisted suicide and euthanasia, including empirical findings.

# PART ONE

---

# Framework and Context

---

# Ethics Goals for Good Care When Patients Face Decisions about Life-Sustaining Treatment or Approach the End of Life

These *Guidelines* concern two groups of adult and pediatric patients: those who face decisions about the use of life-sustaining treatment and care following such decisions, and those who are near the end of life, whether or not a decision about life-sustaining treatment is being considered. These two groups overlap, but are not the same.

Patients who are considering whether to forgo a life-sustaining treatment may be nearer the end of life as the consequence of this decision. However, these patients need not be "actively" or "imminently" dying at the time of a decision. In some cases, a patient may die shortly after a treatment decision is implemented, as when a treatment compensates for an organ system necessary for life. In other cases, a patient's life expectancy is uncertain as a progressive disease process follows its course. Patients who are nearing the end of life may have used life-sustaining treatment and subsequently decided to forgo treatment, or they may be dying of a condition for which there is no effective treatment.

All of these patients face decisions about whether to use interventions that may delay death and about what treatment and care are consistent with their values and preferences. Clinicians caring for these patients must help them cope with their condition and navigate these decisions, assuring good care as these patients near death. These *Guidelines* aim to support clinicians and their institutions in fulfilling these responsibilities. The *Guidelines* are built on ten ethics goals for professionals responsible for the care of adult and pediatric patients who are facing decisions about the use of life-sustaining treatment or who are approaching the end of life, as well as for institutions that provide end-of-life care or make relevant policy. Part One, Section 1 describes these goals. Part One, Section 2 describes nine practical, skills-based ethics competencies that follow from these goals. Professionals who provide care to patients facing treatment decisions or approaching the end of life should make sure they have mastered these competencies. Institutions that provide care near the end of life should make these competencies priorities in ethics education. As some of these competencies may also be relevant to other health care workers (such as paraprofessional aides) who provide care near the end of life, institutions should identify opportunities to include these workers in ethics education. Part One, Section 3 identifies the organizational systems that support these goals and competencies. Part One, Section 4 provides an overview of the social, regulatory, and legal contexts in which care near the end of life is delivered and in which these goals should be pursued and these competencies developed.

## Summary of ethics goals

Goal 1: Relieve suffering.
Goal 2: Respect the experience of living and support the process of dying.
Goal 3: Promote well-being.
Goal 4: Respect persons.
Goal 5: Respect dignity.
Goal 6: Respect relationships.
Goal 7: Respect difference.
Goal 8: Promote equity.
Goal 9: Preserve professional ethical integrity.
Goal 10: Use organizational systems to support good care and ethical practice.

Each of these goals is important. Taken together, these goals describe the practices and structures that offer a compassionate and competent response to illness, fragility, and mortality. The order in which the goals are listed reflects the patient-centered focus of these *Guidelines*, beginning with goals that concern the patient's health, identity, and relationships, and moving outward to goals that concern the policy and processes that support the delivery of good care. These *Guidelines* place considerable weight on the goal of respect for persons, exercised through practices and structures that allow patients to make their own decisions and be confident that these decisions will be honored. The *Guidelines* also recognize that the range of options available to any individual patient is not limitless.

## Description of ethics goals

Goal 1: Relieve suffering. Prevent and alleviate pain and symptoms whenever possible.

Medical progress tends to be measured through advances in the prevention and cure of disease. In the care of persons near the end of life, medicine's traditional emphases on doing no harm and acting to relieve suffering remain the ethical touchstones. Because the relief of suffering should be central to good health care, pain and symptom management and other modalities for the relief of suffering should be fully integrated into health care delivery, including care near the end of life. As some persons who are near the end of life are still pursuing treatment, there is no inconsistency between "therapeutic" and "palliative" treatments, nor can professions and specialties be divided between "curing" or "caring."

Goal 2: Respect the experience of living while supporting the process of dying. Provide persons who are likely to be near the end of life with opportunities for positive experiences and meaning during the remainder of their lives. Offer a supportive and peaceful environment during the dying process to patients and loved ones.

To respect a life is to support the quality of that life to its end. Caring for persons who are likely to be near the end of life is always simultaneously the care of living persons. Supporting the living person requires health care professionals to find out how this person wants to live out his or her life, to collaborate with this person to identify goals of care that reflect and do not conflict with the person's wishes and preferences, and to refine these goals as conditions change. Supporting the person who is nearing the end of life includes providing a peaceful environment and helping this person to discern what is meaningful to him or her.

Goal 3: Promote well-being. Define well-being in terms of patients' goals and values. Prevent avoidable harms, meet the needs and promote the interests of patients, and aim to ensure that the benefits of treatments outweigh their burdens as experienced by patients.

All medical treatments carry burdens. Patients may experience burdens in the form of poorly managed pain and symptoms or treatment side effects, or through the time consumed by treatment-related appointments, or through out-of-pocket treatment expenses. Poorly coordinated care and the health consequences of mistakes or nosocomial infections are other potential treatment-related burdens. These burdens are added to the physical and psychological burdens of living with a life-threatening disease or condition. Because any intervention has the potential to add to a patient's burdens, no treatment option should be characterized as or considered harmless. A patient who faces a decision about life-sustaining treatment or is approaching the end of life can be significantly harmed if life becomes consumed by interventions that are more burdensome than beneficial. While patients, loved ones, or professionals may perceive the possibility of prolonging life as a potential benefit of continuing treatment, extending the length of life is not an ethical imperative in and of itself, regardless of how young or how old a patient is. Each treatment decision should be guided by patient preferences and well-being. Decisions about treatment should aim to ensure that the burdens of treatment do not outweigh their potential benefits from the patient's perspective.

Goal 4: Respect persons. Support and promote patient self-determination. Treat all patients as persons deserving respect.

We respect persons by recognizing their freedom to make choices in accordance with their own values. When health care professionals respect the rights of the individual patient, they demonstrate respect for persons. The courts have recognized that individuals have a legal right to refuse unwanted medical treatment, even if that refusal shortens life. Honoring the individual's legal right to refuse or limit treatment is an ethical imperative and an expression of respect for individual self-determination in a free society. Beyond these legal rights, there is broad ethical consensus within and across health care professions that a patient's preferences should guide the identification of the goals of this patient's care, and that the care plan for the patient should reflect these preferences and goals. Respect for persons also recognizes that individuals are social beings who may consider the interests of others when making decisions and who may choose to make decisions in consultation or collaboration with loved ones or with other trusted individuals. Respect for persons further recognizes children and adolescents as individuals who are developing the capacity to make informed choices about their health care and other aspects of their lives; when their preferences can be ascertained, those preferences should help to guide care.

The right to refuse treatment does not establish a right to demand any and all treatment a patient or surrogate chooses. The goal of respect for persons should not be reduced to "do whatever the patient wants," or "do whatever the surrogate thinks the patient would have wanted," because what a patient (or surrogate) wants may involve a treatment with no potential for physiological benefit, such as antibiotics for a virus. A large literature now addresses patient and surrogate demands for treatment with no potential for benefit. These requests are discussed in Part Two, Section 2E ("Making the Decision at Hand").

**Goal 5: Respect dignity. Create the conditions that help a person who is facing a decision about life-sustaining treatment or is nearing the end of life to sustain a sense of identity that is meaningful and satisfying to that person.**

Caring for a person who is facing a decision about life-sustaining treatment or is approaching the end of life requires close attention to the dignity of the individual—to his or her status as a person and a subject of respect and moral worth. Decisions about life-sustaining treatment may come at a time of physical fragility and can be stressful, challenging a person to determine their guiding values and preferences. For patients near the end of life, the physical and in some cases cognitive deterioration that accompanies terminal illness can pose terrible assaults on the patient's sense of self. By treating individual patients with respect and by organizing care so it helps patients to sustain their identity as persons as their health conditions change and they become more dependent on others, health care professionals help patients to maintain their dignity.

**Goal 6: Respect relationships. Promote supportive ties to loved ones. Maintain the patient's relationships with health care professionals within and across care settings to prevent isolation and abandonment.**

These ethics goals are realized within the context of interpersonal relationships involving the patient, the patient's loved ones, and those responsible for the patient's health care. Promoting autonomy and respecting relationships are compatible goals.

Autonomy means "self-rule," not "self-isolation." Respecting a patient as a person means respecting this person's relationships and supporting a patient's ability to draw on these relationships in making decisions and approaching the end of life. Respecting a patient's relationships and the social context in which the patient has lived his or her life also means supporting those people whom the patient has chosen to be part of his or her current life. Some patients are close to their families of origin, while others are not. Health care professionals should not impose their own preconceptions of who the patient's loved ones are and should respect the constellation of loved ones whom this patient has chosen. This includes supporting the patient's surrogate decision-maker, the loved ones involved in the patient's care, and other caregivers who may be essential to ensuring a patient's well-being by giving them respect and emotional support and by offering them privacy.

Health care professionals must be aware of the potential for conflict among individuals who stand in different relationships to the patient and may have different opinions concerning the treatment decision a patient or a patient's surrogate should make. Disagreements may arise among health care professionals, or between health care professionals and the patient or a patient's loved ones, or among loved ones. Health care professionals should expect that, on occasion, they will need to resolve disagreements. They should have confidence that their institution will provide them with the training and organizational systems to do so. (See the Introduction, note 2, for an explanation of how these *Guidelines* use the term "family." See also Part One, Section 4A ["Social Context"], page 26.)

Goal 7: Respect difference. Acknowledge the role that beliefs, religious commitments, family traditions, and cultural values may play near the end of life and in the lives of individual patients.

America is a culturally diverse society that is continually reshaped by immigration and mobility. Health care institutions and health care professionals serve diverse patient populations. Caring for patients as persons and as social beings requires health care professionals to recognize how personal values and expectations concerning health care may be informed by sources such as beliefs, religious commitments, a family's history and traditions, or a patient's identification with values that the patient associates with an ethnic, racial, or cultural affiliation. Health care professionals should work to understand and respect how an individual's experience of illness and the end of life may be informed by traditions, practices, and beliefs that the patient finds meaningful. As with a patient's personal relationships, health care professionals should not impose their own preconceptions about a patient's beliefs, religious commitments, traditions, or cultural values based on their own past experiences with other patients. Health care professionals should also recognize that distrust of the health care system and personal experience of health disparities may inform how patients and loved ones approach decision-making about life-sustaining treatments and end-of-life care.

Goal 8: Promote equity. Use fair and transparent processes and avoid "bedside rationing."

For nearly every condition, medical treatment options can delay the moment of death. Assuring fairness in access to life-sustaining treatment and to good end-of-life care, and transparency in decisions about such care, is an ethical imperative.

Equity operates on several levels in end-of-life care. At the level of treatment and decision-making for an individual patient, equity requires nondiscrimination. Treatment that is medically indicated for a particular patient should not be withheld by a health care professional on the basis of irrelevant factors such as gender, race, ethnicity, underlying disability, or income level. Also at the individual level, equity requires attention to resource allocation. All health care resources are limited resources. Some health care resources, such as whole blood, transplantable organs, or funds for uncompensated care, are particularly limited. Wasteful practices, including the misuse of resources that have no prospect of benefiting a patient, are not justified, as they direct resources away from patients who may benefit from them. Treatment with no prospect of providing benefit to a patient also imposes burdens on that patient with no justification for doing so.

At the institutional level, institutions have duties to create ethically sound systems for the fair allocation of limited resources and to communicate the rules and procedures to individual professionals and patient care teams. Professionals are responsible for participating in these systems and helping to improve them. However, professionals should refrain from withholding potentially effective interventions at the bedside with the aim of redistributing resources for society. Such decisions are likely to be arbitrary and unfair to patients and ineffective in achieving this aim. Professionals should aim to be effective advocates for their patients by advocating for needed care. Professionals should nonetheless avoid selective advocacy based on factors other than need, as well as "gaming the system" by exploiting loopholes in rules and procedures to divert resources toward some patients. Such steps work against the goal of equity and may also delay the detection and repair of flaws in a system that all patients must rely on.

At the level of institutional policy and broader public policy, the goal of equity is served through efforts to improve decision-making about life-sustaining treatment and end-of-life care. Persons who are ill need more care than persons who are healthy. However, improving end-of-life care requires attention to both the quantity of resources and the quality of outcomes. Providing *better* care to patients facing decisions about life-sustaining treatment and patients nearing the end of life requires using evidence to evaluate the success or failure of specific interventions. It also requires using care planning processes to clarify treatment-related values and preferences in order to guide treatment decisions.

**Goal 9: Preserve professional ethical integrity.** Recognize health care professionals' duty of care and address barriers to good care, such as moral distress and legal myths. Clarify the circumstances in which it is or is not permissible for a professional or institution to withdraw from a case and transfer the duty of care.

Health care professionals have stringent ethical obligations to patients. These obligations are grounded in a duty of care, which prohibits professionals from abandoning patients and requires them to meet standards of care and honor patients' rights.

An institution's policy and processes should recognize that on occasion a health care professional may ask to withdraw from a case on religious or other moral grounds (conscientious objection). Institutions should aim to accommodate this request without compromising standards of professional care and the rights of patients, and while holding the professional responsible for maintaining his or her duty of care by assisting in the orderly transfer of the patient to another professional. Conscientious objection by individual professionals is discussed further in Part Two, Section 2I ("Conflicts and Challenges Related to Treatment Decision-Making").

When a health care institution itself does not provide specific services on religious or other moral grounds, this information should be clearly communicated to patients, surrogates, and loved ones before admission. If an already admitted patient or surrogate makes a care decision that conflicts with institutional limits, the institution should make sure to provide care appropriate for this patient while seeking the orderly transfer of the patient to another institution. In some situations, transfer may not be possible. Judicial resolution of such conflicts may be needed. Conscientious objection by institutions is discussed further in Part Two, Section 6G ("Guidelines on Conflict Resolution").

Health care professionals' ethical integrity can also be challenged by moral distress: situations in which they feel uneasy about a treatment decision or care plan or perceive themselves as complicit in wrongdoing. Moral distress and related disagreements among members of a patient care team have the potential to undermine patient care. Institutions should be alert to the potential for moral distress when decisions are made about life-sustaining treatment and in end-of-life care, offer professionals opportunities to discuss the conditions that may contribute to such distress, and help teams to resolve related conflicts. Moral distress is discussed further in Part Three, Section 3G.

Confusion over what constitutes good practice and the circulation of misinformation can also undermine professional integrity and result in actions that do not serve the interests of patients. Myths about the law—incorrect beliefs represented and circulated as facts—are a persistent problem. These legal myths often reflect fears about professional and organizational liability and are associated with situations involving the withholding or withdrawing of life-sustaining treatment, the use of opioids, or demands for treatment with no potential for benefit. Myths are no substitute for clear, accurate, and current information about the law and about ethical conduct in patient care.

Professionals may also be unclear on how to proceed, ethically and in keeping with the law, when a patient who lacks decision-making capacity has treatment directives that include wishes that do not match the clinical situation at hand, or when working with a surrogate who has been relatively uninvolved in a patient's care. Institutions should provide clear guidance concerning these common and foreseeable scenarios.

Efforts to address the goal of preserving professional integrity through the use of ethics education should include opportunities for health care professionals to discuss their beliefs and concerns about specific problems in patient care and attention to the educational needs of paraprofessional health care workers, as they also seek to act with integrity.

Goal 10: Use organizational systems to support good care and ethical practice. Invest in advance care planning, palliative care services, and ethics services. Establish policy and processes for care transitions. Promote safety, quality, and collaboration within and across end-of-life care settings.

In health care, organizational ethics refers to the policies and processes that help ensure that an institution acts ethically and respects the rights and interests of its patients. When an institution's policies and processes for patient care are soundly conceived, clearly explained, and regularly reviewed, health care professionals can rely on them. When an institution's business decisions are ethically sound, these decisions are seen to be consistent with the institution's obligations to its patients, and to the understanding that health care is a social good. Policies and processes create structures to support good care, such as advance care planning, palliative care services, ethics consultation and education services, and discharge planning. These structures support the decision-making processes described in these *Guidelines*. They should be integrated into institutional systems for patient safety and quality improvement to ensure that the safety of patients and the quality of the care they receive are addressed at the organizational, as well as the clinical, level.

Organizational ethics addresses not only single institutions, but also collaboration among institutions caring for overlapping patient populations. Recognizing these institutions as having related concerns supports innovations such as portable medical orders and facilitates the identification and resolution of care problems that travel with patients when they transfer between care settings.

# Ethics Education Competencies for Health Care Professionals Caring for Patients Facing Decisions about Life-Sustaining Treatment or Approaching the End of Life

These *Guidelines* refer frequently to the "responsible professional," meaning the medical professional in charge of a patient's care for a given care episode or in a particular care setting. All physicians who may be responsible at some point for the care of patients facing decisions about life-sustaining treatment or patients nearing the end of life must be ethically competent to function in this role. In some settings the "responsible professional" may be a nurse or a physician-nurse duo.

These *Guidelines* propose nine ethics competencies that reflect professional consensus on the practices that promote sound outcomes in treatment decision-making and in end-of-life care. They are summarized here to support the use of these *Guidelines* among professionals who care for patients facing decisions about life-sustaining treatment or nearing the end of life. These patients rely on many different professionals, so responsibility for good care should be shared among professions, specialties, and care settings.

All health care professionals who care for patients facing decisions about life-sustaining treatment and patients nearing the end of life should recognize their responsibility to master these aspects of their practice. Institutions should offer educational programs designed to help professionals master these competencies. Institutions should also ensure that institutional policy and processes support good practice across all settings in which patients facing decisions about life-sustaining treatment or nearing the end of life receive treatment and care.

The Bibliography supporting the Introduction and Part One includes a selection of published literature and web-based research and educational materials that can support clinician education on these competencies. The selected references for each topical section of the *Guidelines* include empirical studies, critical analyses, and model processes that can also support clinician education.

Competency 1: Maintain current knowledge of practice recommendations and research findings on life-sustaining treatment and end-of-life interventions.

The professional should know how to find and use current professional guidance on decision-making concerning life-sustaining treatment and end-of-life interventions relevant to the professional's specialty or care setting. The professional should also be up to date on pertinent research findings and practice recommendations. Clinician education offering opportunities to discuss and reflect on professional guidance and related research and recommendations can support this competency. For selections from the research and professional literatures, see the Bibliography supporting Part Two, Section 4 ("Guidelines for Care Transitions") and Part Three, Section 4B ("Decision-Making Concerning Specific Treatments and Technologies").

Competency 2: Learn how to integrate pain and symptom management into all treatment plans in all care settings for patients of all ages and into discharge plans.

The professional should know how to manage pain and symptoms arising from the patient's disease or condition and its treatment or from decisions to forgo treatment. The professional should also know how to consult and collaborate with palliative care specialists as needed. Institutional investment in palliative care services and professional training, as well as institutional policies and processes for palliative care consultations, can support this competency.

Competency 3: Learn how to elicit patients' treatment-related values and preferences, establish and document goals of care, and develop care plans that reflect these preferences.

The professional should know how to communicate with patients to elicit their preferences and plan care. Institutional processes for advance care planning and for the preparation and use of care plans for seriously ill patients of all ages support this competency.

Competency 4: Learn how to collaborate with patients and surrogates and work with loved ones during treatment discussions and decision-making.

The professional should learn techniques for effective communication with patients, surrogates, and loved ones. The professional should be expert at discussing the benefits and burdens of starting, continuing, or forgoing specific interventions. Education that includes training in communicating with a range of adult and pediatric patients, with surrogates, with other loved ones, and across cultures supports this competency. Institutional hiring of bilingual staff and staff who are familiar with the different cultures reflected in patient populations, as well as clinician access to certified health care interpreters (including sign language interpreters) and to speech-language pathologists skilled in communicating with nonverbal or hearing-impaired patients, also support this competency.

Competency 5: Learn how to collaborate with other professionals during treatment discussions and decision-making, in the process of transfer, and in discharge planning.

The professional should know how to manage the flow of information among professionals involved in a patient's care, to maintain continuity of care and ongoing communications with patients and loved ones across shifts and care settings. The professional should also know how to air different clinical perspectives within patient care teams and collaborate to resolve care problems. Ethics education and institutional processes for documenting treatment decisions and for transferring information during care transitions support this competency.

Competency 6: Learn about the common causes of distress experienced by patients, surrogates, loved ones, professionals, and staff in end-of-life care settings, and how distress may affect treatment decision-making and the delivery of care.

The professional should be able to recognize the signs of psychological, spiritual, existential, or moral distress experienced by patients and others when treatment decisions are being made and in as patients approach the end of life, and should be familiar with methods for responding to different types of distress. Ethics education, ethics consultation, palliative care consultation, and institutional investment in mental health, spiritual care, and social work services support this competency.

Competency 7: Learn how disagreements arise in decision-making about life-sustaining treatment and in care near the end of life and how to prevent and resolve conflicts with patients, among loved ones, and among professionals.

The professional should be familiar with common and less common sources of disagreement and conflict and should know how to initiate and participate in conflict resolution. Ethics consultation, ethics education, and institutional conflict-resolution processes support this competency.

Competency 8: Learn how to recognize legal myths about decisions concerning life-sustaining treatment and end-of-life care and take responsibility for correcting misinformation.

The professional should have accurate knowledge of federal and state law and policy concerning advance directives, treatment decision-making with patients and surrogates, pain and symptom palliation, and other aspects of care for patients facing decisions about life-sustaining treatment and patients nearing the end of life. The professional should be capable of identifying incorrect assertions about the law. The professional should also take responsibility for correcting misinformation and for drawing attention to practices that are informed by these myths rather than by accurate knowledge. Ethics education in collaboration with institutional legal counsel and risk management supports this competency.

Competency 9: Develop personal capacity for ethical reflection and participate in opportunities to explore ethical concerns arising in decisions about life-sustaining treatment and care near the end of life.

Practices of reflection on the caregiving process and on treatment decisions are integral to the care of patients facing decisions about life-sustaining treatment and patients who are near the end of life. The professional should be offered and should seek out regular opportunities to discuss and learn from complex cases and to explore the impact of caregiving on caregivers themselves. The professional should also participate in the development of ethically sound policies and processes. Institutional investment in an ethics service that offers opportunities for reflection and the development of ethics education supports this competency.

# Organizational Systems Supporting Good Care and Ethical Practice

The quality of end-of-life care, and care for patients facing decisions about life-sustaining treatment, relies on organizational systems as well as the knowledge, skills, and integrity of individual health care professionals. Even well-designed systems alter over time, as institutions grow, their patient population changes, or they adapt to new economic realities. Research into system failure shows that poor results can often be traced to design flaws and the accommodation of known flaws, rather than to individual bad actors. This means that system design in health care has ethical dimensions.

Health care delivery is complex. Systems for health care delivery should be constructed to deliver results that support the ethical aims of medicine and ethically competent practice by health care professionals. For example, participation in an organization's patient safety systems, such as its methods for preventing medication errors, should be recognized as a means of promoting patient well-being. Clinician education should include opportunities to think critically about the organizational systems in which clinicians routinely participate and to improve these systems by proposing and testing innovations.

Health care leaders can have a profound influence on systems for health care delivery. Leaders are responsible for establishing and communicating institutional priorities. This means that the leaders of any institution that provides care for patients facing decisions about life-sustaining treatment or patients nearing the end of life should embrace the ethical goals described in these *Guidelines*. Efforts to improve the quality of care for these patients will benefit from health care leaders who see end-of-life care as part of health care, rather than a failure of health care.

Part Two, Section 6 of these *Guidelines* offers guidelines on the institutional policies and processes for decision-making about life-sustaining treatment and care near the end of life. These policies and processes cover ethics consultation and other ethics services, palliative care consultation, advance care planning, continuity of care, conflict resolution, and the role of legal counsel and risk management in clarifying law and policy. The following systems are among those that can also support the goals and competencies described in these *Guidelines*.

## Patient safety

All patients, including patients facing decisions about life-sustaining treatment or patients nearing the end of life, can suffer injuries through harms associated with particular interventions, medication errors, nosocomial infections, the progressive impact of comorbid conditions, and errors associated with miscommunication and other discontinuities of care. Patient safety mechanisms such as "near miss" reporting can identify areas of care where safety can be improved. Capital improvements such as the redesign of facilities to prevent falls or to reduce infections associated with shared rooms may significantly contribute to the safety of patients facing decisions about life-sustaining treatment and patients nearing the end of life who may be vulnerable to falls and respiratory infections, while creating a safer environment for all patients.

## Information technology

Accurate and accessible documentation is integral to care planning, treatment decision-making, and the transfer of information between professionals involved in a patient's care. Information technology also offers opportunities to monitor patients' health outcomes, to guide future care, and to identify whether certain patients are receiving poor care.

## Health communications directed to patients and the public

An institution's website, intranet, and other communication resources are tools for sharing information about policy and processes related to end-of-life decision-making and care. Using these tools effectively supports informed decision-making and fair process.

## Quality improvement

Quality in health care requires attention to research, models, and standards for clinical decision-making about life-sustaining treatment and end-of-life care. Evidence-based interventions, including clinical practice improvements supported by "checklist"-type tools, can be developed and used in these settings. An institution's human resources systems also should include quality improvement mechanisms, such as processes for evaluating staff performance, incentives and opportunities for staff to improve skills relevant to the care they provide, and ways of acknowledging and rewarding outstanding performance.

Institutions vary in the extent to which they systematically evaluate the quality of their performance in the care of patients facing decision-making about life-sustaining treatment and patients who are near the end of life. The Bibliography includes a selection of literature and web-based resources relevant to quality assessment and improvement.

# Social, Economic, and Legal Contexts

## A. Social Context

A health care professional who enters a patient's life when this patient is facing decisions about life-sustaining treatment or care near the end of life must be prepared to establish a trusting relationship quickly, as decisions about life-sustaining treatment and goals of care may need to be made rapidly. This situation is familiar to professionals who work in acute-care settings. Changes in a patient's condition can also affect a long-standing relationship between a patient and a professional that was established with the goal of curing or managing disease long-term. As the goals of care shift, this professional will need to clarify new goals and the patient's preferences for life-sustaining treatment and end-of-life care.

A professional should expect that the discussion of a patient's values and preferences will be informed by this person's history and relationships inside and outside of health care systems.

### Decision-making experiences

Individuals come to decisions about end-of-life care with different decision-making styles and histories. Before making major decisions, some persons seek out all the facts themselves. Others rely on loved ones or a trusted individual, such as a personal physician, attorney, clergyperson, colleague, or mentor. Some individuals enjoy making decisions, while others do not. A person's lifelong approach to decision-making will influence how he or she approaches decisions about life-sustaining treatment. Some persons, well before the end of their own lives, have had experience in medical decision-making; others have had little experience. During the course of a long, progressive illness, a person's approach to decision-making may undergo shifts. This person may value exercising self-determination at some times, while at other times may prefer to delegate decision-making to others.

Persons who have lived with stable or slowly progressing disabilities for years may be especially experienced in making medical decisions and may have made many decisions about life-sustaining treatment throughout their lives. By contrast, a person who has been newly diagnosed with a life-threatening disease may be shocked by the possibility of being near the end of life and may resist any discussion of end-of-life treatment preferences and goals. This patient needs support from professionals who know how to conduct these discussions and who can help the patient and loved ones involved in the patient's care to come to terms with the diagnosis and prognosis.

## Relationships

Relationships are an important aspect of social context. As the end of a person's life nears, there are usually loved ones present. Professionals caring for persons near the end of life should be prepared to work with different constellations of loved ones, not limited to those defined by biological or legal relationship to the patient. "Family," as this term is used in these *Guidelines*, may include close friends or an intimate partner whose relationship to the person may or may not be recognized by law. It may include a relative, friend, or paid caregiver who serves as the patient's designated care partner by accompanying the patient to treatment and helping the patient to coordinate care. It may include the patient's appointed health proxy or surrogate decision-maker. The family may include individuals who love the sick person deeply and individuals who detest this person, or individuals immobilized by the circumstances or their emotions. It may include someone who does not want the sick person to die, and someone who wishes this person dead sooner rather than later. In these *Guidelines*, the words "family" and "loved ones" cover this range of relationships. Professionals caring for persons near the end of life should expect to work with loved ones.

Some persons are alone at the end of life, by choice or circumstance. Elderly hospitalized patients and nursing home residents who are without any family or social relationships (often called "unbefriended") may have been socially isolated for many years.[6] If these patients have decision-making capacity, they should be encouraged to consider appointing a health proxy or naming a surrogate and to document any preferences concerning treatment. They should be assisted and supported in doing both of these things. If these patients decline to designate a surrogate and then lose decision-making capacity, the professionals who care for them will need to trigger an institutional process to put a surrogate decision-maker in place. It may also be necessary to seek judicial appointment of a surrogate. (See Part Two, Section 2D, "Surrogate Decision-Making.")

## Social identity and affiliations

A patient's social identity may include values, beliefs, and practices associated with his or her cultural affiliations, religious commitments, family traditions, or personal interests, or a combination of these and other factors. These identifications may influence how a person approaches decisions about life-sustaining treatment and end-of-life care. However, individuals are always more than group representatives. A health care professional may know or may observe that certain health-related values, beliefs, and practices are associated with a particular social group. However, the professional cannot infer any individual patient's values and preferences concerning treatment based on the professional's knowledge of a group, knowledge that itself may be faulty or incomplete. If a patient or a patient's loved ones indicate that certain social identifications are important to them, professionals should work to learn what those identifications mean to the patient in particular, and how those identifications can be respected in decisions about life-sustaining treatment and end-of-life care.

Patients or loved ones who have experienced discrimination or a lack of access to health care, or have witnessed this within a group with which they identify, may believe that their lives are not valued by health care professionals. These experiences, observations, and beliefs may lead patients to conclude that opting for more treatment will protect them against neglect or ensure that they receive better quality health care. It is important to address these concerns directly to provide needed and truthful reassurance.

## Disability

Many people who have lived with a disability have had significant experience with the use of life-sustaining treatments and technologies. If a person with such experience is diagnosed with a different and potentially life-threatening condition or faces the progression of a long-term condition, professionals involved in this person's care should work to understand this person's views on the use of life-sustaining treatments and technologies in the current circumstances. Communication concerning life-sustaining treatments in the context of disability is discussed in detail in Part Three, Section 2.

## Aging

Decisions near the end of life are often associated with diseases of aging, and so are likely to be affected by an individual's age and experience of aging. Great leaps in life expectancy during the twentieth century mean that Americans now expect to age over decades and may try to delay the onset of serious disease into the eighth, ninth, or tenth decade of life. However, support for living long when a person is in fragile health may be hard to find. The aging individual's life experience may be reduced to being a patient, with the risk that the exercise of self-determination will be narrowed to medical decision-making. Professionals caring for aged patients are likely to be younger than their patients, as are the adult children who frequently serve as surrogates or family caregivers. Professionals and family caregivers alike may be tempted to rely on generalizations and stereotypes about "the elderly." It is always important to determine and respond to the values and preferences of the aged person as an individual. As health care professionals who provide end-of-life care frequently care for aged patients, ethics education should aim to include perspectives from professionals with expertise in geriatric medicine, nursing, mental health, and social work. These professionals can contribute insights into aging as a process that is not limited to the diseases of aging and into the challenges aging persons face as their health changes or deteriorates.

## B. Economic Context

### The cost of care as a burden near the end of life

Persons facing decisions about potentially expensive life-sustaining treatment or those nearing the end of life may be particularly vulnerable to burdens associated with the cost of health care in the United States. They may be confronting or incurring significant medical expenses not fully covered (or not covered at all) by insurance. Their capacity for work and their income may be reduced, if they are not already on a fixed income. Seriously ill persons may struggle to manage and pay for their own care, even if some of their care is paid for by federal or state programs such as Medicare and Medicaid or by private insurance. Implementation of the Patient Protection and Affordable Care Act of 2010 at the federal and state levels should reduce the number of patients who lack access to health insurance or who are underinsured. However, life-sustaining treatment and care near the end of life may also impose economic burdens on loved ones if they must cover unreimbursed expenses or lose household income to become unpaid caregivers.

Health care professionals responsible for discussing treatment options with patients and loved ones may find it challenging to ask about the potential financial burdens associated with various options. Patients and loved ones themselves may be unsure whether it is appropriate to ask about the cost of treatment or to factor this into decision-making. Professionals aware of the high cost of specific therapies may struggle with how—or whether—to present treatment options that are medically appropriate but that a patient or loved ones would have to pay for themselves, or how to present costly interventions that are likely to offer only marginal benefit. They may be uncertain whether policy reforms aiming at increasing access to health insurance will reduce these inequities or have any effect on the cost of care.

Addressing cost, especially if patients or loved ones express concern about cost, is a legitimate part of the decision-making process. However, health care professionals should be cautious about assuming what insurance plans and entitlement programs will or will not cover, or what patients or loved ones can afford. Discussing openly the costs of treatment options and involving others within the institution who are expert in payment options can avoid mistaken assumptions. A patient or loved one may need information and counseling about insurance, entitlements, or charitable programs that may cover or reduce the cost of care.

All institutions that provide care to patients facing decisions about life-sustaining treatment or patients nearing the end of life should work toward transparency and consistency in institutional policies and practices concerning cost. Institutional leaders should support the ability of professionals—in particular, physicians, nurses, and social workers—to understand cost as an ethical issue in the delivery of health care and to communicate effectively with patients and loved ones concerning the cost of treatment options. To support these aims, these *Guidelines* include a discussion guide for institutions (Part Three, Section 5) on resource allocation and the cost of care as issues of equity. This discussion guide is designed for use in ethics education and to support institutional policy-making.

## Hospitals

According to the Centers for Disease Control and Prevention, approximately 2.5 million individuals die in the United States each year.[7] Of these individuals, approximately 50 percent die in hospitals.[8] These deaths may include patients who died shortly after transfer from a nursing home or other care setting.

Each hospital is its own miniature society whose customs are familiar to its hundreds or thousands of workers but remain foreign to most patients and their loved ones. One of the realities that patients and their loved ones may not know about hospitals is how profoundly hospitals are shaped by economics. The typical patient near the end of life is old enough to qualify for Medicare, and so will have health insurance coverage. Under the Medicare system, however, hospitals (and outpatient providers) currently are not directly reimbursed for services having to do with communication, care planning, and many aspects of palliative care, but rather for treating a patient's specific diseases and related symptoms. As a result, there are powerful financial incentives for hospitals to define care in terms of reimbursable treatment interventions and diagnostic testing, to prioritize quantity of care over quality of care, and to set a lower value on patient services that are not income-generating. These incentives have a large role in shaping the delivery of end-of-life care in hospitals but may be poorly understood by health care professionals themselves, as well as by patients and loved ones.

## Nursing homes

Nursing homes are the setting for approximately 20 percent of total deaths in the United States each year.[9] They are even more strongly influenced by Medicare and Medicaid reimbursements and regulations than are hospitals and may be reimbursed at lower levels than hospitals for caring for individuals with similar or even higher levels of impairment. Nursing homes may transfer residents to hospitals for care episodes for a number of reasons, including a practice of shifting the cost of caring for very sick residents to hospitals until death occurs or Medicare will no longer cover hospitalization. Nursing home medical directors and nursing directors should be familiar with models for delivering cost-effective palliative care in the nursing home setting, to reduce hospital transfers and allow residents to die in place. Part Two, Section 4B ("Guidelines on Care Transitions for Nursing Home Residents") and the Bibliography supporting that section include further discussion and citations concerning this topic.

## Hospice programs

Hospice programs, which provide care for approximately 40 percent of all patients who die in the United States each year (including hospice services delivered in hospitals, nursing homes, and other settings, in addition to private homes), are also influenced by Medicare and Medicaid reimbursements.[10] An adult patient becomes eligible for Medicare-covered hospice care (the Medicare Hospice Benefit) once a physician certifies that the patient is terminally ill with a life expectancy of six months or less if the terminal disease process follows its normal course. A patient who elects to enroll in hospice and to forgo further life-sustaining treatment aimed at cure or long-term survival is covered under the Hospice Benefit, which reimburses hospice programs for medical, nursing, social work, and other palliative care services provided by an interdisciplinary team of hospice professionals and trained volunteers. Within the scope of hospice services, a patient may temporarily revoke his or her hospice election to receive treatment that is consistent with the patient's goals of care and palliative care plan but is not offered by a particular hospice program.

Children receiving hospice services may be covered by their parents' private insurance or by the Medicaid Hospice Benefit, which is offered by nearly every state. Private insurance plans vary in the scope of hospice services covered but often cover the full range of hospice services, funding them on a per diem basis.

Parents or guardians of some dying children may find it difficult to decide to forgo curative treatment completely. In recognition of this reality, the Patient Protection and Affordable Care Act of 2010 (Section 2302) requires states to offer "concurrent care for children" under Medicaid and the Children's Health Insurance Program (CHIP, formerly known as SCHIP). Under this provision, children who qualify for hospice care can receive hospice services concurrently with curative treatment. For example, a child with advanced cancer would be able to receive hospice care at home while continuing to receive radiation as an outpatient.

### Chronic disease and end-of-life care

Mortality data reveal that most deaths in the United States result from chronic progressive diseases, including diseases affecting the functioning of major organ systems, cancer, and physical deterioration caused by worsening frailty and dementia.[11] Chronic progressive diseases that may gradually impair a person for years before death can add burdens at the end of life. For example, patients with Alzheimer's disease, the most common form of dementia, may live with progressively worsening dementia for years or even decades and may also develop chronic comorbid conditions associated with aging. Hospitalizations and other care transitions to treat comorbid conditions can be disorienting for patients with underlying dementia. Chronic progressive conditions may also create economic and other burdens for loved ones who provide unpaid care or cover unreimbursed home care costs. Patients who have lived with chronic illnesses may have had difficulty obtaining pain and symptom management, mental health care, and specialized palliative care services available to hospitalized patients with similar diagnoses. Chronic disease often leads to end-of-life care, and efforts to improve the quality of chronic care will improve the quality of end-of-life care.

## C. State and Federal Context

State and federal constitutions, statutes, regulations, policies, and court decisions affect end-of-life care, as do health care professionals' knowledge and beliefs about the law. Good care can be derailed by misinformation or misplaced fears about law and legal liability. In addition, some well-intentioned laws and policies may introduce rather than prevent problems in health care. For these reasons, ethics education on decisions about life-sustaining treatment and care near the end of life must be attentive to the relevant legal and regulatory framework in the United States and in a particular state. Educators in clinical settings should work to assure good quality information about the law, not only through formal advice from institutional counsel and risk management, but also through informal sources such as supervisors, colleagues, and the staff grapevine.

### Medicare, Medicaid, and the states

Most individuals who die in the United States each year are Medicare-eligible, due to their age, or because they make use of the Medicare Hospice Benefit. Some are also on Medicaid, due to low income or disability, or because they "spent down" their assets to qualify for Medicaid coverage for long-term care. While Medicare is shaped largely by federal rules, Medicaid is fifty different systems jointly financed by the federal government and each state, which administers its own program within federal guidelines that allow for considerable latitude. End-of-life care that may be funded by Medicaid includes pediatric hospice care, as well as nonhospice care provided to residents of long-term care facilities.

### State law and treatment decision-making

Both federal and state law secure the rights of individuals to make decisions about life-sustaining treatment and end-of-life care. These rights are protected by federal and state constitutions, the federal Patient Self-Determination Act, state statutes, and federal and state judicial decisions. Federal and state law similarly address the rights of individuals to use advance directives to guide their care and treatment decision-making if they lose decision-making capacity in the future. Both federal and state law assure that individuals do not lose the right to make decisions about their care if and when they lose the capacity to decide for themselves; instead, a surrogate makes decisions on the patient's behalf under standards governed by state law within parameters set by federal constitutional law. Most states also have statutes or court decisions on the determination of death. All have regulations that are applicable to health care institutions where decisions are made about life-sustaining treatment and where care near the end of life is provided. Two states (Oregon and Washington) have statutes that authorize a process for physician-assisted suicide under certain conditions, while a third state (Montana) has a court decision that appears to allow some physician-assisted suicide. (See Introduction.)

As noted, misinformation about the law on life-sustaining treatment and end-of-life care may circulate among health care professionals and workers, including administrators, clinicians, and paraprofessionals such as nurses' aides. For example, physicians and nurses caring for patients facing decisions about life-sustaining treatment or patients nearing the end of life may have a faulty understanding of the legal authority of surrogates, or may be reluctant to use doses of opioids adequate to manage a patient's pain because of a belief that administering opioids is legally risky. Administrators may believe, incorrectly, that health care advance directives must be documented in a form recommended by state statute to have any effect. In all these cases, misinformation will compromise good care and hamper progress toward ethics goals.

Law and ethics are interrelated but not the same. Health care professionals and institutions have both ethical and legal responsibilities toward the patients in their care. Federal and state law on life-sustaining treatment and end-of-life care can be ethically problematic. For example, highly detailed statutory requirements for advance directives can be confusing to patients and professionals alike and pose barriers to honoring patient choices.[12] Similarly, the development and authorization of portable medical orders designed for use by clinicians across care settings may be hampered by various existing state laws and regulations.[13] As legal concerns over life-sustaining treatment and end-of-life care can derail good care, these *Guidelines* include recommendations for institutional legal counsel and risk managers (Part Two, Section 6F).

These *Guidelines* do not offer legal advice; for that, clinicians and administrators should turn to their legal counsel. Instead, they focus on describing and encouraging ethically competent care. Law should support ethical practice, and for the most part, it does. Evolving practices in end-of-life care may require legal changes, policy reforms, or both.

# PART TWO

Guidelines on Care Planning
and Decision-Making

---

# Guidelines for Advance Care Planning and Advance Directives: Using Patient Preferences to Establish Goals of Care and Develop the Care Plan

These *Guidelines* address not only those patients immediately facing decisions about life-sustaining treatment and those nearing the end of life, but also the broader population of patients planning ahead about life-sustaining treatment and end-of-life care. Most individuals have preferences concerning their current and future treatment and care. These preferences, and the values underlying them, vary from person to person. The ethical standards for surrogate decision-making (see Part Two, Section 2D) for a patient who does not currently have decision-making capacity call for health care professionals to follow the explicit preferences, written or oral, which this patient articulated prior to losing decision-making capacity. A patient's directions may include the designation of a surrogate decision-maker. The patient can appoint an individual as surrogate (also known as a proxy, health proxy, or health agent) through the completion of a written document (such as a durable power of attorney for health care, also known as a "proxy directive") or in a treatment directive or "living will," which also states treatment preferences. The patient can also identify a surrogate, state treatment preferences, or both, in oral instructions. In some health care facilities, a patient who wishes to choose (or limit) which other individuals can visit or receive information about this patient during a hospitalization can also complete a "hospital visitation directive."

When patients lose the capacity to make their own medical decisions without having provided treatment directions and stated explicit preferences, the ethical standards for surrogate decision-making call for the surrogate to infer what the patient probably would have wished from knowledge of and experience with the patient. However, when there are no explicit preferences from the patient, the surrogate and loved ones have less guidance about what the patient would have wanted. They may disagree with one another or with the patient's physician about what to do. Many cases that are referred for ethics consultations result from conflicts over decision-making for patients who currently lack the capacity to make their own medical decisions and who did not leave instructions while they had decision-making capacity.

These *Guidelines* recommend advance care planning. Asking patients about their values and preferences, and documenting and using these preferences, is integral to good care and ethically sound practice.

A professional responsible for the care of patients, especially those facing or considering decisions about life-sustaining treatment or end-of-life care, should know how to initiate advance care planning with the patient and how to use documents and oral instructions resulting from this process.

The term "advance care planning" describes a process (which ideally includes the completion of advance directives) that is initiated by a patient or a health care provider and designed to achieve three goals:

1.  **To elicit a patient's values and preferences concerning future treatment and record the patient's treatment preferences**

A patient's values and preferences for life-sustaining treatment and end-of-life care can guide the patient's medical treatment and how this patient completes his or her life. Patients may assume that a physician or other health care professional will initiate this discussion, or patients themselves may raise the subject. Offering a patient who has been diagnosed with a progressive or life-threatening disease, or who is expected to face decisions about life-sustaining treatment, the option of participating in advance care planning will often be welcomed, though some patients may prefer not to participate. The first step in the advance care planning process is a discussion or interview. The patient completes this step in collaboration with a physician, nurse, or other health care professional. If desired by the patient, loved ones may also participate. The outcomes of this discussion may include, but should not be limited to, the completion of advance directives, portable medical orders, or both. Those documents record the patient's treatment preferences as well as the patient's preferred surrogate if the patient loses decision-making capacity in the future.

Even if a patient does not wish to complete any advance directives, the advance care planning process gives the patient an opportunity to discuss values, preferences, and goals related to treatment and care and to have specific wishes and preferences documented in the medical record so they are known to health care professionals. The use of a structured advance care planning process is recommended in adult and pediatric care settings to ensure that information provided by patients is appropriately documented and integrated into medical records to guide medical care. For descriptions of advance care planning processes, see the portion of the Bibliography supporting this section.

**2.   To use a patient's values and preferences to establish goals of future care, often in light of a patient's established diagnosis, prognosis, and treatment options**

Some patients are interested in providing guidance for future care if they should lose decision-making capacity, even though they have no diagnosis as yet. This advance care planning should be encouraged. For these patients, establishing goals of care refers to the application of a patient's values and preferences to a range of possible future medical circumstances. For patients who have already received a diagnosis of a potentially life-threatening condition or have a condition that is progressing, advance care planning is more concrete. When a patient begins advance care planning after diagnosis or progression, the discussion of the patient's values and preferences is likely to encompass goals related to this condition and its treatment. Sometimes patients need help clarifying their goals. For example, a patient whose values include prolonging life, perhaps expressed in terms of self-identity ("I'm a fighter"), or who harbors a specific hope ("I want to see my granddaughter graduate from college next spring") may also hold preferences that include limiting hospitalizations (perhaps expressed as "staying out of the hospital" or "remaining at home with my family"). This patient will need a discussion to clarify these potentially conflicting preferences and to establish goals of future care that can accommodate these values and preferences.

**3.   To develop a future care plan that reflects a patient's preferences and goals, and to modify the care plan so it remains consistent with changes in goals**

When patients have identified their treatment preferences and what changes in circumstances would make them alter their goals and this information has been memorialized in advance directives or the medical record or both, professionals are able to consult this information to create care plans that fit with the patient's choices. Advance care planning helps professionals, surrogates, and loved ones to use previously identified patient preferences to guide care after a patient has lost decision-making capacity. The structure provided by an advance care planning process can also help health care professionals work with patients who still have decision-making capacity but whose prognosis has changed due to disease progression, requiring a review of the patient's preferences for future care.

Ideally, advance care planning should be completed while a patient is still reasonably healthy and in the outpatient setting, although in some cases it will be necessary to initiate advance care planning following an illness episode or during hospitalization. Professionals in primary care relationships with patients should make a practice of discussing treatment preferences and of offering information about the option of completing advance directives in advance of hospitalization or a serious decline in health. The diagnosis of a progressive disease or life-threatening condition in a patient of any age should be one trigger for initiating an advance care planning process—if possible, after an adjustment period so the patient has time to consider the probable future course of the disease. Not every patient will want to discuss future choices, particularly if the patient's immediate goal is the cure or control of disease. However, introducing the concept of goals of care, and the idea that treatment options should be considered in light of whether they help the patient to achieve those goals, establishes an ethical framework for discussions of how care should be guided in the future, including in the event the patient loses the capacity to make his or her own decisions.

The professional who is best situated to conduct advance care planning may be the patient's primary care provider or a specialist physician responsible for the patient's treatment following diagnosis, such as an oncologist or cardiologist. Nonphysicians, such as nurses, social workers, or professional (board-certified) chaplains, may share responsibility with physicians for advance care planning.[14] Whenever possible, the physician responsible for the patient's care should be involved in the process to make sure the physician understands the patient's preferences and is prepared to honor them. Advance care planning that includes the preparation of portable medical orders (see Part Two, Section 4) requires the involvement of a professional authorized to sign this type of document.

If advance care planning must be initiated while a patient is hospitalized, the professional responsible for the patient's care during the hospitalization is responsible for initiating advance care planning, unless an institution conducts advance care planning through another mechanism, such as a palliative care consultation.

The patient should be encouraged (but not required) to include his or her appointed or intended surrogate in the advance care planning process, so that the surrogate also understands the patient's preferences and is prepared to honor them.

Part Two, Section 2 of these *Guidelines*, on treatment decision-making, can be used as a basic model for conducting advance care planning with a patient who has decision-making capacity.

Health care professionals should encourage patients with decision-making capacity to appoint or designate a surrogate decision-maker if they have not already done so. Health care professionals should encourage patients to discuss their preferences with their appointed or designated surrogates.

Advance directives help meet the needs of patients who lose decision-making capacity near the end of life. All patients, apart from those who have *never* had decision-making capacity and require different surrogacy arrangements (described in Part Two, Section 2D, "Surrogate Decision-Making," on surrogacy for adult patients who have never had decision-making capacity, and in Part Two, Section 3, on surrogacy for children), should have access to the benefits of advance directives, as they are authorized in all states and serve as a means of protecting patients' rights under the federal Constitution and the federal Patient Self-Determination Act, as well as under state constitutions and statutes. It is especially useful for patients to designate a future surrogate decision-maker in the event the patient loses decision-making capacity. When a treatment directive does not cover the treatment decision at hand or includes multiple directions that seem to conflict with one another, a surrogate can strive to decide as the patient would wish. Encouraging a patient to designate a surrogate, to state their treatment preferences, and to discuss those preferences with their surrogate promotes good care.

**Care planning should include opportunities for patients to review their advance directives periodically to determine if they reflect the patient's current wishes and preferences.**

If a patient's existing directives do not address the actual medical situation the patient now faces, the professional responsible for advance care planning should assist the patient in updating or revising existing directives. This review and discussion also gives the professional an opportunity to ask the patient if the surrogate named in the patient's directives has been made aware of the patient's wish that this person serve as surrogate. The professional should also check to ensure that existing advance directives and any updates to these directives are properly integrated into medical records.

**Advance care planning with a seriously ill patient should aim to document preferences relevant to foreseeable medical emergencies and decisions to guide care across care settings.**

Portable medical orders provide emergency medical personnel and other health care providers with explicit guidance concerning future medical contingencies that are likely due to the current condition of a seriously ill or frail and debilitated patient. This documentation accompanies a patient across care settings, including home, hospital, nursing home, and hospice. A set of portable medical orders is often referred to as a "POLST" if it is based on the Physician Orders for Life-Sustaining Treatment (POLST) Paradigm. (See Part Two, Section 4C, "Guidelines on Portable Medical Orders.") Portable medical orders help assure that emergency medical personnel and staff in any new care setting will be apprised of existing advance directives and care preferences.

**Advance care planning for a patient who is likely to be near the end of life should address how the patient wishes to spend his or her remaining life.**

When a patient is forgoing life-sustaining treatment, or the patient's underlying disease is inexorably progressing and the patient is likely to be nearing the end of life, the responsible health care professional should make sure to clarify the patient's preferences about how he or she wishes to spend the remainder of his or her life. This is especially important as patients may lose decision-making capacity near the end of life. These *Guidelines* recommend that professionals initiate these shared deliberations well before the onset of a medical crisis, if possible, and while the patient still has decision-making capacity, to identify care and treatment preferences, including where the patient prefers to spend the remainder of his or her life. This requires discussion of what setting the patient prefers (be it home or another setting), whether that preference is realistic, and what can be done to try to accommodate the patient's preference (for example, by helping the patient and loved ones to identify hospice programs that can set up services in the home).

**Professionals should receive appropriate training in advance care planning, including the proper use of advance directives and portable medical orders in different care settings.**

Advance care planning and successful use of advance directives involves collaboration among different health care providers, including the professional responsible for a patient's care, and other professionals and paraprofessionals responsible for the delivery of care. All of these health care providers should be trained in the proper use of the documents and orders created through advance care planning.

This training should identify common misconceptions that create barriers to advance care planning. For example, if a patient, loved one, or health care professional believes—incorrectly—that advance care planning is only for patients who wish to forgo treatment or who are near the end of life, the person who holds this belief may conclude that it is premature to discuss advance care planning when a patient is relatively healthy or accepting treatment. Training should clarify, and institutional processes should reinforce, that advance care planning is appropriate for anyone who seeks to plan for possible loss of decision-making capacity, including temporary loss of decision-making capacity in a medical crisis. Advance care planning is also important for a patient whose relationship with an intimate partner may or may not be recognized by law.

Ethics education for health care personnel concerning advance care planning should include attention to how successful educational efforts have been structured elsewhere. Three models for advance care planning that incorporate professional education and that may be broadly relevant in the care of elderly patients or in large patient populations in the United States are *Respecting Choices, EPEC (Education in Palliative and End-of-Life Care) for Veterans* and *ELNEC (End-of-Life Nursing Education and Consortium) for Veterans*, and the Alzheimer's Association advance care planning services and educational materials.

*Respecting Choices* is an advance care planning program developed by Gundersen Lutheran Health System.[15] Studies of this replicable model have found that an advance care planning process that includes community outreach, professional education, and institutional collaboration leads to high levels of interest and participation among community residents and that the resulting documentation is likely to be integrated into participants' medical records. A selection of studies of *Respecting Choices* is included in the Bibliography supporting Part Two, Section 1.

*EPEC for Veterans* and *ELNEC for Veterans* are professional education curricula on treatment decision-making and end-of-life care that include advance care planning models for use in any setting in which veterans of the U.S. military receive health care.[16] These curricula describe the potential relevance of a veteran's dates of service and combat history (the details of which may be unknown to loved ones) to the patient's preferences and concerns about life-sustaining treatment and care near the end of life and provide guidance to professionals in sensitively addressing combat history in advance care planning discussions and documentation. As many veterans receive some or all of their health care outside of the Veterans Health Administration system, all professionals who care for veterans in any health care setting should be aware of these professional education resources.

The Alzheimer's Association offers extensive advance care planning services and educational materials through its toll-free twenty-four/seven helpline, public website, and local chapters.[17] All professionals who care for patients diagnosed with progressive forms of dementia, in any setting, should be familiar with these readily accessible resources and should share this information with patients, surrogates, and loved ones. As persons who have been diagnosed with progressive forms of dementia may retain decision-making capacity at the early stage of this disease, patients with early-stage dementia should be offered opportunities to learn about and participate in advance care planning.

The Bibliography supporting this section includes selections from the extensive empirical literature on advance care planning. The websites included in the Bibliography provide additional resources, including links to the models described above.

# Guidelines for the Decision-Making Process

## Introduction: Communication and the Decision-Making Process

This section of these *Guidelines* describes a decision-making process that is grounded in the goals described in Part One. All of these goals are relevant to any treatment decision presented to patients (or their surrogates) who are facing decisions about life-sustaining treatment and patients who are near the end of life.

Effective communication among health care professionals, patients, and surrogates is integral to informed decision-making near the end of life. The health care professional responsible for a patient's care should support informed decision-making by taking these steps:

- Collaborate with the patient to establish goals of care that reflect patient preferences for treatment and care in light of the patient's diagnosis, prognosis, and current condition. If the patient lacks decision-making capacity, the professional should work with the patient's surrogate to establish the goals of care in keeping with the standards for surrogate decision-making addressed in Part Two, Section 2D ("Surrogate Decision-Making").
- Explain each treatment decision in the context of the patient's goals of care and as part of a care plan that at all times provides for palliative care.
- Allow sufficient time and social support for decision-making deliberations.
- Share current clinical information, in clear language, with the patient and surrogate (if any) and other loved ones as appropriate, and among team members.
- Describe treatment options, including the option to forgo particular interventions, and the consequences of each option. Treatment options may include the option to take no action, defer a decision, or conduct a time-limited trial of a treatment.

- Document treatment decisions so they are clear and available to all team members.
- Regularly review treatment decisions with the patient and, if the patient lacks decision-making capacity, with the surrogate.

For additional guidance concerning communication with patients and surrogates about treatment decisions, see Part Three, Sections 1, 2, 3, and 4.

# The Decision-Making Process

## A. Evaluating the Patient

It is essential that an identified health care professional have primary responsibility for a patient's care and for supporting informed decision-making. This decision-making requires effective communication with the patient or surrogate, if any.

The likelihood that a patient who may be near the end of life will move among care settings means that the responsible health care professional may not be the same person throughout the course of a patient's final illness. If there is more than one physician involved in a patient's care, the patient, loved ones, other professionals, and even the physicians themselves may be uncertain about "who's in charge." The rapid growth in the number of general internists working as hospitalists means that hospitalized adult patients are increasingly likely to be cared for by physicians who are not their primary care providers. (This trend also affects pediatric care, as some hospitalists are pediatricians.) Patients in academic medical centers are also likely to be cared for by a series of physicians as residents rotate on and off shifts. To prevent confusion, a physician (or, in some settings, a physician-nurse duo) should be designated as being the responsible health care professional and thus have primary responsibility for a patient's care. This information should be communicated to the patient, surrogate, loved ones, and team members.

The responsible health care professional should evaluate the patient's condition as a necessary foundation for any decision about life-sustaining treatment and care near the end of life.

The first person to recognize that a patient's condition may have changed or deteriorated, prompting a new or renewed need to discuss treatment options, may be someone other than the responsible health care professional, such as a nurse, a home health aide, a loved one, or the patient. Those working or living closely with the patient are often the first to recognize increasing debilitation, lack of responsiveness to treatment, or other signs of change, as well as any emerging concerns of the patient. They may also be the first to observe that the patient (or surrogate) is considering whether to forgo treatment. It is important to communicate these changes to the responsible professional, to trigger an evaluation of the patient's concerns and condition.

The responsible professional should perform the clinical evaluation of the patient's concerns and clinical condition in consultation with other members of the care team. As the clinical evaluation is the beginning of decision-making deliberations, it may include loved ones or others involved in the patient's care if their involvement is acceptable to the patient. The responsible professional conducting the evaluation should respect the patient's right to prevent the disclosure of health information to other persons.

If it has already been established that the patient does not have decision-making capacity or if the patient's decision-making capacity is fluctuating, the patient's surrogate should be made aware of the evaluation. The responsible professional and the patient should also confer directly, as long as the patient is capable of doing so. The patient without full decision-making capacity may still be able to comprehend what the professional has to say and may be able to understand that an evaluation is being undertaken to aid decision-making. For additional guidance on decision-making involving patients without full decision-making capacity, see Part Two, Section 3, and Part Three, Section 2.

The goal of the evaluation is to yield the following information:

### 1. The patient's current concerns
This is the starting point of any evaluation. Understanding the patient's concerns focuses the responsible professional's evaluation by clarifying the concerns and changes that may have triggered the evaluation.

### 2. The patient's diagnosis
Confirming the diagnosis will help clarify relevant treatment options. However, the responsible professional should not routinely subject the patient to burdensome testing to confirm the diagnosis, but should, in consultation with the patient or surrogate, determine how much more certainty is needed to permit the patient or surrogate to make an informed decision about treatment.

### 3. The patient's prognosis
Understanding the patient's likely course with or without life-sustaining treatment is important for decisions about treatment and care near the end of life. While the responsible professional may not be able to say exactly how much longer the patient will live, the professional should be able to describe likely outcomes.

### 4. The treatment options, their likely benefits and burdens for the patient, the likely effects of each option on the patient's prognosis, and the professional's recommendation, if any, within the context of the patient's goals of care, care plan, and known preferences
The responsible professional should address all treatment options that have potential for benefiting the patient, including the option to forgo medical treatment. If the responsible professional believes that a particular option is most closely aligned with the patient's goals

of care, this recommendation should be made clear to the patient or surrogate. However, all relevant treatment options, including the option to forgo treatment, should be addressed.

5. **The patient's capacity to understand the current diagnosis, prognosis, treatment options, and treatment recommendation, if any**

Patients are presumed to have decision-making capacity unless health care professionals perform an evaluation yielding the clinical conclusion that the patient now lacks this capacity or a court determines that the patient lacks decision-making capacity. (See Part Two, Section 2B, "Determining Decision-Making Capacity," below for detail on determining decision-making capacity as part of the evaluation.)

The evaluation is also an opportunity for the responsible professional to confirm whether the patient has previously expressed and documented treatment preferences through an advance care planning process, an advance directive, or other means. Preferences expressed in advance directives (and/or noted in the medical record) to guide care after the loss of decision-making capacity become effective after the loss of decision-making capacity and so do not supersede the decisions of a currently competent patient.

Evaluation should be an ongoing part of patient care, with reevaluation whenever the patient's concerns, preferences, or condition changes.

## B. Determining Decision-Making Capacity

If there is a significant question about the patient's capacity to make treatment decisions, the responsible professional should assess the patient's decision-making capacity.

### "Competence" and "capacity"

The terms "competence" and "capacity" (and their opposites, "incompetence" and "lack of decision-making capacity") are often confused with one another. Traditionally, the term "incompetent" has referred to a person who had been determined by a court to lack competence (adjudication of incompetence), while the phrase "lack of decision-making capacity" has referred to a person who has been determined by a health care professional (usually a physician, and often a psychiatrist) to lack the capacity to make health care decisions. Beginning in the 1990s, many states revised their relevant statutes and replaced the competence/incompetence terminology formerly reserved for the legal context with the capacity/lack of capacity terminology formerly reserved for the clinical context. As a result, it is no longer possible to make a clear distinction between the terms "competence" and "capacity" as these terms are used in health law and health care in the United States. The terminology of "capacity" is now likely to be used in both contexts.

More important than terminology is the question of who has the authority to decide that a patient lacks decision-making capacity, so that a surrogate decision-making process must be used. Although courts have the authority to declare individuals to lack decision-making capacity either generally or for a specific purpose (such as medical decision-making or handling financial affairs), a health care professional has the author-ity to make a clinical determination of a patient's capacity to make medical and other health care decisions. It is important to consult legal counsel and/or local law concerning the legal effect of a clinical determination of decision-making capacity and the need for further legal process.

### Clinical determination of decision-making capacity

A patient has decision-making capacity when the patient has the ability to:

1. understand his or her condition and treatment options;
2. deliberate in accordance with his or her own values and goals and make an unco-erced decision among treatment options; and
3. communicate (verbally or nonverbally) this decision.

A patient with decision-making capacity should be an active participant in the decision-making process concerning his or her own care unless he or she chooses not to do so. Therefore, a patient with decision-making capacity should not have life-sustaining or other medical treatment initiated or withdrawn without his or her informed consent. The only exception is an emergency situation in which the patient is temporarily unable to give consent and any relevant decisions this patient has already made are unknown to per-sonnel responding to the emergency. In those circumstances, there is generally a presump-tion of patient consent to life-saving treatment. To prevent situations in which seriously ill patients receive emergency treatment that is inconsistent with their prior decisions, these *Guidelines* describe and recommend the use of medical orders that document patient deci-sions concerning foreseeable emergencies and are authorized for use by emergency medical personnel and across care settings. (See Part Two, Section 4C, "Guidelines on Portable Medical Orders.")

As noted, patients are legally presumed to have the capacity to make treatment deci-sions unless it is determined, through clinical evaluation or judicial decision (or both, when needed), that they currently lack it. Clinicians must act in accordance with this presump-tion of capacity. A patient need not have decision-making capacity for all purposes to have the capacity to make the treatment decision at hand. Some patients have the capacity to make one type of decision, but not another.

If a patient is determined to lack decision-making capacity, the responsible profes-sional should inform the patient of this, and that a surrogate will exercise decision-making authority. (See Part Two, Section 2D, "Surrogate Decision-Making," below.) The pro-fessional should make every effort to support the patient's continued involvement in decision-making, even if the surrogate makes the ultimate decision. Respect for persons, including persons without decision-making capacity, means that patients who can par-ticipate in making decisions about their own care should be encouraged to do so. In the event that the patient regains decision-making capacity, the responsible professional should promptly acknowledge both this and the patient's renewed decision-making authority.

A patient should be able to challenge a determination concerning capacity or incapacity to make treatment decisions.

If the patient objects to a determination that he or she lacks decision-making capacity, the responsible professional should seek an ethics consultation. Review by the institution's ethics consultation service, ethics committee, or other mechanism should be prompt. If possible, no treatment decision should be made until the challenge has been resolved. If a treatment decision must be made in the interest of the patient's well-being, the patient should be assumed to have decision-making capacity until the challenge is resolved. Some cases may need judicial resolution.

## C. Identifying the Key Decision-Maker

The responsible professional needs to know who the key decision-maker is with respect to a patient's treatment decisions.

The responsible professional should start with the assumption that the key decision-maker is the patient, who may choose to consult with family members or other loved ones in making decisions. If the patient does not have decision-making capacity concerning health care decisions, a surrogate must serve as the key decision-maker. (See D, "Surrogate Decision-Making," below.)

## D. Surrogate Decision-Making

### Identifying the surrogate

When a patient is determined to lack decision-making capacity, the responsible professional should determine whether the patient has designated a surrogate decision-maker or has a court-appointed surrogate. If no surrogate has been appointed or designated, the responsible professional should determine whether there is an appropriate surrogate who is able to make treatment decisions in accordance with the patient's values and preferences.

There are several ways in which surrogates may be designated, appointed, or identified:

### Surrogate designated by patient

If the patient has appointed a surrogate for health care decision-making through a durable power of attorney for health care or, absent such a document, has designated a surrogate through any other written or oral statement, that person serves as the patient's surrogate decision-maker. An advance directive in which a patient designates a surrogate may also be known as a "proxy directive." Terms such as "proxy," "health proxy," "agent," or "health agent" may be used in institutional policy or in statutes to refer to a specific individual designated by a patient as his or her surrogate.

As described in Part Two, Section 1, these *Guidelines* recommend that health care professionals encourage patients with decision-making capacity both to designate a surrogate and to discuss their wishes and treatment preferences with the surrogate as well as with the responsible professional. Documenting these preferences while the patient still has decision-making capacity can help guide and support surrogate decision-making later.

### Court-appointed surrogate

If the patient has not designated a surrogate but a court has appointed a surrogate for the patient (known as a "guardian," or in some states, a "conservator") and the treatment decision is within that person's authority, then that person serves as surrogate.

### Identification of default surrogate with reference to statute

Some states have laws stating a priority order for designating adults eligible to serve as surrogates if there is neither a surrogate designated by the patient nor a court-appointed surrogate. For adult patients, the hierarchy is often spouse or legally recognized domestic (civil) partner, then adult child, then parent, then sibling. Health care professionals should consult the law of the state in which they practice. The eligibility of a patient's same-sex spouse, civil partner, or other intimate partner to serve as a surrogate if there is neither a surrogate designated by the patient nor a court-appointed surrogate should be recognized. States currently differ in their legal recognition of these relationships in their default surrogate-selection statutes and also in their recognition of close friends in these statutes. Proxy directives are particularly important for patients who wish to designate their intimate partner or have a close friend serve as their surrogate decision-maker.

### Multiple potential surrogates

Occasionally, a patient's designated surrogate may not be able or willing to take on this responsibility, or there may be more than one eligible surrogate, or there may be tension between the named surrogate and another person close to the patient. Advance directives that designate but do not rank multiple surrogates can present similar problems. In situations such as these, the responsible professional will need to work with the patient's loved ones to determine how decisions consistent with the patient's explicit preferences—or (if those are not known) the patient's values and preferences inferred from past knowledge of or experience with the patient, or (if those, too, are unknown) the patient's best interests— will be made by an individual surrogate or through collaboration between a surrogate and others close to the patient. In those states that have statutes governing the appointment of surrogates, the statute may contain provisions for the resolution of such cases. In some cases, judicial resolution may be needed.

## Surrogacy for pediatric patients

The usual surrogate for a minor is a parent or guardian. As conflicts may arise between parents or guardians, between the surrogate and an adolescent patient, or between the surrogate and another family member, responsible professionals should be aware of the special considerations related to surrogate decision-making in pediatric care settings. (See Part Two, Section 3.)

## Surrogacy for adult patients who have never had decision-making capacity

Adult patients who have never had decision-making capacity, perhaps due to long-standing cognitive or psychiatric disabilities, may have surrogacy arrangements in place or may need such arrangements. Professionals responsible for the medical care of adult patients who have never had decision-making capacity should make sure that such arrangements are in place. Some states have statutes requiring the judicial appointment of a guardian for an adult patient who has never had decision-making capacity. Other states have mechanisms for surrogate decision-making committees composed of appointed and trained volunteers to make medical decisions on behalf of residents of state-regulated facilities who lack decision-making capacity and also lack other surrogates. Professionals should be aware of any legal requirements for the judicial resolution of decision-making disputes concerning the care of adult patients who have never had decision-making capacity and of the existence of any surrogate decision-making program in the state in which they practice.

Concerns or conflicts may arise when an adult patient who has never had decision-making capacity can express some preferences, and these preferences differ from a surrogate's perception of this patient's best interests. Health care professionals may be able to help a surrogate for an adult who has never had decision-making capacity to better understand how the benefits and burdens of treatment are being or would be experienced by this person. Involving such patients in collaborative decision-making, if they are willing and able to do so, and consulting with the caregivers of such patients may support surrogate decision-making. This situation may call for ethics consultation and in some cases judicial resolution.

For additional guidance on communication with patients whose disabilities affect cognition, see Part Three, Section 2.

## Uninvolved surrogates

Working with any surrogate who has agreed to serve in this role but has not been involved in the patient's life may be challenging for the professional responsible for the patient's care. If a professional is concerned that a surrogate is not sufficiently familiar with the patient's values and preferences or does not have sufficient knowledge of or experience with the patient to make treatment decisions, the professional should seek ethics consultation. This situation also may require legal consultation. The professional may need to work with the uninvolved surrogate to make decisions that are in keeping with the patient's explicit preferences; or, if these are not known, the patient's inferred values and preferences; or, if none of this is known, the patient's best interests.

## Surrogacy arrangements for "unbefriended" patients

Institutional policy and processes should provide clear guidance to professionals on how to proceed when caring for a patient without decision-making capacity who lacks a surrogate. The Veterans Health Administration's detailed and transparent process may serve as a model for other institutions.[18] The VHA's surrogate decision-making process describes how the responsible professional, other members of the health care team, an existing or appointed ethics committee, and a facility's senior leadership should collaborate when a patient without decision-making capacity lacks a surrogate and a treatment decision is at hand. The VHA process also provides guidance to professionals on how to collaborate with legal counsel to petition for a court-appointed guardian with authority to make health care decisions for a patient who lacks decision-making capacity and also lacks a surrogate. This measure protects the patient's rights by ensuring that a recognized surrogate is in place for health care decisions, including those about life-sustaining treatment.

Having the responsible health care professional unilaterally make decisions for an "unbefriended" patient is an unsatisfactory approach. Such a practice compromises patient autonomy by leaving decisions in the hands of an individual (or a series of individuals across shifts) who cannot devote singular focus to the question of the patient's explicit preferences, inferred values and preferences, or best interests relevant to this decision. It also compromises transparency, as there is no review and accountability for the decision that the professional makes unilaterally. Waiting until the patient's medical condition worsens into an emergency so that consent to treat is implied is another unsatisfactory way to deal with this problem, as it compromises patient care by waiting for a crisis and allows no orderly consideration of the patient's explicit preferences, inferred values and preferences, or best interests, or of the option to forgo what is now emergency treatment.

## Clarifying identity of surrogate

The responsible professional should make sure that the name of a patient's surrogate or a description of any other surrogacy arrangement appears in the patient's health records so that this information is available to all members of the health care team. The responsible professional should check that family members or other loved ones involved in a patient's care are aware of the identity of the designated surrogate, unless the patient has given instructions that this information not be shared. Confusion and tension may arise when family members do not know who the surrogate is, make an incorrect assumption about the surrogate's identity, or are unaware of treatment decisions being made by a surrogate who is not present at the patient's bedside.

## Standards for surrogate decision-making

A surrogate for a patient without decision-making capacity should follow the three-tiered standard for surrogate decision-making. The responsible professional should describe these standards to the surrogate and to any other individuals involved in decision-making. Adhering to these standards ensures that a surrogate's decision will honor the patient's explicit preferences, or, if these are unknown, the patient's inferred values and preferences, and if these too are unknown, the patient's best interests.

In making decisions, the surrogate should apply the following standards in this sequential order of priority:

### 1. Patient's directions

The surrogate follows the patient's treatment directives or other explicit preferences, written or oral.

### 2. Substituted judgment

If there are no treatment directives or other explicit preferences allowing the use of the first standard, the surrogate bases decisions on the patient's inferred values and preferences, as best they can be gleaned from knowledge of and experience with the patient.

### 3. Best interests

If there are no treatment directives or other explicit preferences from the patient and the surrogate lacks enough information to use the second standard, the surrogate should choose the treatment option that will be in the patient's best interests in light of the patient's condition, prognosis, and treatment options. When the patient is an incapacitated adult, this is sometimes explained as choosing what a "reasonable person" would choose if in the patient's circumstances. (Best interests decision-making in pediatric care settings, in which parents or guardians usually serve as surrogate decision-makers, is discussed in further detail in Part Two, Section 3.)

Making treatment decisions on behalf of a person without a directive or even information about what this person would want can be challenging to professionals and surrogates alike. When framing the goal of best interests decision-making on behalf of a patient, it is helpful to clarify that a decision in a patient's best interests is one that considers how a person, in these circumstances, would probably wish to be treated. The application of the best interests standard will therefore consider:

- what this patient is experiencing, including his or her pain or other symptoms, suffering, and experience of receiving treatment, plus his or her understanding of the health condition and the purpose of treatment;
- the ethical imperative to relieve suffering, both physical and psychological;

- what *most but not all* patients experience as treatment "benefits" or treatment "burdens" (for examples, see Part Two, Section 2E, "Making the Decision at Hand," below);
- the uniqueness of this patient as an individual;
- the treatment options with some realistic potential for benefiting this patient;
- the benefits and burdens of each of these treatment options, including the option to forgo further life-sustaining interventions; and
- other values that a reasonable person in the patient's circumstances would wish to consider, were this person able to do so.

The situation of a patient who has lost decision-making capacity and has dementia or other irreversible neurological deterioration may present a special challenge in surrogate decision-making. If the prior expressed preferences of this patient now appear to conflict with the best interests of this patient in his or her current condition, the health care professional may be uncertain whether the patient's prior expressed preferences should take priority over what appear to be the patient's current best interests. Ethics consultation may be necessary in such cases. Advance care planning with patients with early-stage dementia, using processes developed for these patients to clearly specify their future treatment preferences, is recommended to honor patients' rights and prevent future care problems. (See Part Two, Section 1.)

### The patient with fluctuating decision-making capacity

In some patients, decision-making capacity may fluctuate. For example, some patients have decision-making capacity at certain times of the day, but not at other times. Reversible causes of incapacity may include fatigue, metabolic factors, overmedication, undertreatment of pain, or delirium induced by the stress of hospitalization. If a patient with fluctuating decision-making capacity has a surrogate and the patient and surrogate agree on a treatment decision, the decision should be implemented. If this patient and the surrogate do not agree on this decision, the responsible professional should seek to resolve uncertainty about the patient's decision-making capacity. If it is possible to postpone a treatment decision and adjust conditions so that the patient regains capacity, the decision should be postponed. If the patient regains decision-making capacity, then the guidelines for a patient with decision-making apply and the patient makes the decision. If the patient does not regain decision-making capacity and it is no longer possible to postpone the decision further, the guidelines for a patient without decision-making capacity apply and the surrogate makes the decision. In view of the disagreement between the patient and the surrogate about this decision, the responsible professional and the surrogate should discuss which treatment option is most compatible with the patient's explicit preferences (if known), inferred values and preferences (if the surrogate can ascertain these), or best interests. Ethics consultation may be needed.

## E. Making the Decision at Hand

In presenting a treatment decision to a patient or surrogate, the responsible professional should review the patient's goals of care, including any treatment preferences already reflected in the care plan, and describe how the decision at hand relates to these preferences and goals.

In making the treatment decision, a patient with decision-making capacity will weigh relative benefits and burdens among treatment options. Individuals differ in their perceptions of benefits and burdens and in how they balance them. For *most but not all* patients, consequences of treatment that are experienced as benefits include:

- the relief of pain and/or symptoms that cause suffering;
- improved functioning;
- the opportunity to live longer, if the quality of prolonged life is acceptable to the individual patient;
- the opportunity to do things that have meaning or give pleasure to the patient; and
- the possibility of fulfilling specific goals.

For *most but not all* patients, consequences of treatment that are experienced as burdens include:

- pain and/or symptoms that result in suffering;
- the perception or prospect of cognitive impairment, helplessness, or loss of self;
- diminished ability to do things that have meaning or give pleasure to the patient; and
- financial cost or other stress imposed on the patient or on loved ones.

For additional guidance on assessing benefits and burdens associated with specific treatment options, see Part Three, Section 4.

Members of a patient's health care team should at all times make clear to patients and loved ones that palliative care is part of good care and can be provided with any treatment option, including the option to forgo life-sustaining treatment. The health care team should make sure that pain and symptom management and access to other palliative care services are continuously available to patients.

Requiring patients and surrogates to repeatedly request relief for pain and symptoms is contrary to the ethical goals of these *Guidelines*. This practice is not in keeping with current standards of pain management and is unnecessarily burdensome for patients and disruptive for loved ones. These *Guidelines* recommend that palliative care be integrated into the care of all patients so patients and surrogates can make treatment decisions—including but not limited to decisions near the end of life—confident that they will have continuous pain and symptom management and access to other palliative care services, such as mental health services, social services, and chaplaincy services. Patients or surrogates may need to make specific treatment decisions concerning the benefits and burdens of various palliative care options.

As all health care professionals have a duty to relieve suffering and a patient's surrogate must follow the patient's explicit preferences (if known), inferred values and preferences (if those can be ascertained), or best interests, a surrogate cannot decide that a patient should have no access to pain relief or other palliative care services. Such a decision would not serve the patient and would be contrary to the standards of medical practice.

### Time-limited trials in decision-making

When a patient who is facing decisions about life-sustaining treatment or who is near the end of life, or the surrogate for this patient, expresses a desire to start or forgo a life-sustaining intervention, the responsible professional should ask the patient (or surrogate) why he or she is inclined to make this decision.

This question helps the professional to understand the values and beliefs of the patient, or the surrogate's view of how this decision serves the patient's explicit preferences, inferred values and preferences, or best interests. The dialogue can also reveal why the patient or surrogate is making the decision now and whether the patient or surrogate believes that this is the only opportunity to make a decision about this particular intervention.

**Whenever possible, the responsible professional should offer a patient or surrogate the option of a time-limited trial of the intervention under consideration.**

As a matter of ethics, decisions to start or forgo life-sustaining treatment can be revisited at any time and can be reversed if a patient changes his or her mind, or if the surrogate concludes this is warranted. The use of a time-limited trial may assist a patient or surrogate in assessing the benefits and burdens of an intervention. Time-limited trials are common in some areas of clinical practice, such as pediatrics. (See Part Two, Section 3.)

For guidance on time-limited trials see Part Two, Section 2G ("Implementing the Decision") below. For additional guidance on time-limited trials of specific life-sustaining treatments, see Part Three, Section 4.

**The responsible professional should clarify that a decision about one treatment does not necessarily dictate decisions about other treatments.**

A decision to forgo one kind of life-sustaining treatment does not mean that a patient must forgo all other forms of treatment. For example, patients with do-not-resuscitate (DNR) orders may receive other life-prolonging treatments. The DNR decision means only that cardiopulmonary resuscitation (CPR) will not be attempted if the patient stops breathing or goes into cardiac arrest.

Health care professionals should not use the phrase "doing everything" to represent maximal therapeutic intervention. Professionals should ask and clarify what patients or surrogates mean if they use this phrase.

It is not clear what "doing everything" means. Maximal therapeutic intervention may involve multiple medications and technologies, each carrying burdens. Lumping these interventions into "everything" may mean decision-makers will not be fully informed about burdens and benefits and may undermine a patient's or surrogate's ability to understand that some treatments may no longer be of use. Offering or agreeing to "do everything" to prolong life can prematurely stop discussion, making it difficult to identify and forgo those life-sustaining treatments that offer little or no benefit to a patient or to withdraw treatments once they have ceased to be of benefit.

Asking patients or surrogates if they want "everything" may also be misleading if patients, surrogates, or other loved ones infer that "everything" means better care. The responsible professional should not frame treatment decisions in ways that make patients or families feel that to do less than "everything" is wrong, or that to agree to "everything" is right. Presenting treatment decisions in the context of the patient's current or foreseeable medical problems and the treatment options available to address these problems clarifies the scope of the decision and the nature of potential benefits.

Whatever options for life-sustaining treatment are discussed, the responsible professional should also describe what the health care team will do for the patient to control pain and symptoms and to provide social support. This reassures the patient, surrogate, and other loved ones that the patient will receive good palliative care for the rest of the patient's life, no matter what decisions are made about life-sustaining treatment.

The presentation and discussion of treatments with benefits that include the potential to sustain life should not be reduced to the shorthand of "life-or-death decisions."

Some decisions about life-sustaining treatment are likely to affect the length of a patient's remaining life in that the patient's death may be expected to occur sooner if a decision is made to forgo treatment. However, such decisions do not conclusively determine how long a patient will live, nor do they guarantee that a patient who continues life-sustaining treatment will live longer than a patient with the same condition who stops treatment. In their discussions with patients, and when implementing treatment decisions, health care professionals should avoid the suggestion that a decision about a life-sustaining treatment in the context of terminal illness has a certain ("life or death") outcome, and in particular, that the decision-maker bears the burden of determining how long the patient will live. When a patient is terminally ill, a decision to continue treatment may have some potential to delay the patient's death but cannot reverse an ultimately fatal disease trajectory.

The professional who is explaining the likelihood of benefit from a particular treatment should be aware of the possibility that population-based statistics may be misinterpreted and that decision-makers need to understand both the nature of the benefit and its likelihood. If a patient or loved ones believe that a "10 percent chance of benefit" means that ten out of one hundred patients in this situation are fully cured, this false belief may inform subsequent deliberations and decisions about continuing or ending treatment. If a professional uses an expression such as "one in a million" to express an extremely small likelihood of treatment benefit, the patient or loved ones may well interpret this to mean that, every so often, one patient will be cured.

When discussing the option of hospice enrollment, professionals should be aware that this may sound like a "death" decision to patients and loved ones, and they should be prepared to describe the extent to which hospice patients can continue to receive treatment aimed at symptom relief and improved quality of life while receiving optimal palliative care. As some treatments may be incompatible with hospice, a team member or other health care professional, such as a palliative care specialist, with expert knowledge of available hospice services should be involved in these discussions. For additional guidance concerning discharge to hospice, see Part Two, Section 4D.

The responsible professional should be prepared for questions from the patient or surrogate concerning treatment with no potential for physiological benefit and concerning experimental treatment. The responsible professional should also be prepared for questions about physician-assisted suicide and euthanasia. In all such cases, the professional should take care to clarify terms and to identify and address the underlying issues of particular concern to an individual patient or a surrogate.

### Requests for treatment with no potential for benefit

There is no ethical obligation to offer a patient treatment options that have no possibility to provide physiological benefit relative to the patient's diagnosis, prognosis, and current medical condition. To introduce treatment burdens without possibility of benefit causes harm and misuses resources. Ethics education should support the ability of health care professionals to respond to requests for treatment with no potential for physiological benefit by offering clear explanations of why certain treatments can no longer benefit a patient. Broadly characterizing a treatment as "nonbeneficial" or "futile" should be avoided, as these terms do not explain why a particular treatment would fail to meet a treatment goal. Lawyers and risk managers in health care institutions should clarify that treatment that cannot provide physiological benefit to a patient is not the standard of care, to counteract the belief of some health care professionals that to refuse to provide a requested treatment, even if the treatment has no potential for benefit, is to risk legal exposure for substandard care.

A treatment that cannot provide physiological benefit could potentially offer some psychological benefit to a patient who wants to be "in treatment" or "doing something." However, providing the treatment is ethically problematic, as the responsible professional would be in a position of either withholding the information that would clarify that the treatment is of no physiological benefit or encouraging the patient to hold a false belief by failing to correct a patient's misperception of a treatment's effectiveness. Moreover, such a situation adds burden, no matter what placebo effect or psychological assurance it may offer. In the interests of patient well-being and the fair distribution of limited resources, including limited personnel available for hands-on care, the responsible professional should not use treatment with no potential for physiological benefit in an effort to deliver psychological benefits. The professional should seek to deliver these benefits instead through psychological and palliative care modalities and collaboration with specialists in those areas.

A treatment with small potential for limited physiological benefit should be discussed in the context of the goals of care and with careful attention to the likelihood of benefit, how the potential benefit would be experienced by the patient, and likely or certain burdens. For additional guidance concerning decisions about cancer treatments with small potential for limited benefit, see Part Three, Section 4G.

### Requests for experimental treatment

The responsible professional should be prepared to discuss clinical trials for which a patient may be eligible and should expect that some patients or loved ones will have researched experimental treatments and may seek help in enrolling in trials. When a patient becomes a research subject in a clinical trial or otherwise receives experimental treatment, the potential benefits of the treatment relative to its risks and burdens are as yet unclear. Because any experimental treatment may add some burden, and because such treatment could result in additional suffering for little or no benefit, the responsible professional should take care to explain foreseeable and potential treatment-related harms, and also the uncertainty surrounding experimental treatment. The responsible professional should, in talking with patients and loved ones, be attuned to the possibility of "therapeutic misconception": the belief that an experimental treatment will indeed offer individualized benefits to a research participant. The therapeutic misconception may be more prevalent among patients enrolled in Phase I clinical trials (where benefit is least likely) due to the common misperception that these toxicity trials offer a "last chance" for treatment benefit.

Health care professionals should be mindful of the language they themselves use to characterize experimental treatments, to avoid the suggestion that experimental treatments are "better" or "more advanced" than standard treatments simply because they are newer. If the responsible professional is also a clinical investigator involved in a trial for which the patient is eligible, this professional or another member of the health care team must take care to explain the potential benefits, burdens, and risks of this experimental option, in comparison to the benefits and burdens of nonexperimental treatment options. The professional should ensure that the patient's interests are not superseded by others' research interests and that the patient's decision to enroll in a trial is not influenced by a desire to please the professional who is supervising care. For additional guidance concerning decisions about experimental cancer therapies, see Part Three, Section 4G.

**Requests for physician-assisted suicide or for euthanasia**

A patient with decision-making capacity may ask about physician-assisted suicide, which is allowed in some forms by the law of at least two states, or about euthanasia, which is illegal in the United States. (See Introduction.) Surrogates and other loved ones may also ask about these practices. The responsible professional should take special care to clarify such requests, as it is common for people to confuse these practices with decisions to withhold or withdraw life-sustaining treatments or with the use of medication to relieve pain and symptoms. Ambiguous language can also lead to confusion. A patient or surrogate who asks if there is any way to "get this over with" *may or may not* be asking about PAS or euthanasia. This request may indicate a desire to forgo further life-sustaining treatment, or suggest a need to revisit the patient's palliative care plan in response to the patient's changing needs, or reflect a patient's fear that he or she is becoming a burden to loved ones. The responsible professional or any other team member speaking with the patient or surrogate should take care not to dismiss this inquiry and should clarify the concerns underlying this request.

Professionals should be certain that they themselves understand the ethical distinction between the use of medication with the intent to relieve pain and symptoms (including rare situations in which medication for symptom relief may foreseeably hasten death) and the use of medication with the intent to bring about death. A lack of clarity concerning the distinction between the relief of pain and symptoms and practices such as physician-assisted suicide or euthanasia, or a failure to correct legal misinformation about this distinction, can result in suffering due to undertreated pain and confusion and distress among loved ones and team members. Professionals should therefore be able to explain this distinction clearly to patients, loved ones, and colleagues. For key legal and ethical distinctions, see the Introduction. For additional guidance on palliative sedation to relieve intractable symptoms, see Part Three, Section 4.

Professionals in states where PAS is legal should be familiar with relevant state law and policy and with related organizational policy and procedures.

## F. Documenting the Decision

When a patient or surrogate makes a decision to have a life-sustaining treatment withheld or withdrawn, the responsible professional should document this decision and ensure that the requisite signed orders and any other documentation of this decision are promptly added to the patient's health records.

Documenting decisions about life-sustaining treatment is crucial. Accurate and accessible documentation ensures that all members of the health care team know about the treatment decision and orders, which they must honor. In addition to protecting patient's interests and rights, documentation also protects the interests of everyone involved in making the decision by showing that the decision was the result of an appropriate process, explaining the decision, and allowing for the decision to be reviewed as needed.

Documentation alone does not ensure that patients' decisions concerning life-sustaining treatments and other aspects of care will be honored. A health care institution needs policies and procedures for entering and posting new orders. Members of health care teams responsible for the care of patients facing decisions about life-sustaining treatment or patients nearing the end of life should receive regular training in how to use these orders and documents and how to interpret and follow care plans in the course of caring for a patient. This training should reach personnel on all shifts and should address the fact that some team members will be unfamiliar with their responsibilities with respect to patients' treatment decisions, or may hold mistaken beliefs concerning these responsibilities.

### Documenting decisions about emergency interventions

When a patient or surrogate decides to forgo a life-sustaining emergency intervention such as CPR, the responsible professional should write an order and document the decision so the patient will not receive the unwanted treatment. As noted above, a patient with a DNR order or the surrogate for this patient may choose to continue, start, or forgo other treatments. Patient preferences concerning emergency interventions should be documented in a way that ensures that orders such as DNR are accessible to all medical personnel who may be involved in emergency treatment.

The use of a recognized process for creating and using portable medical orders effective across different care settings (see Part Two, Section 4) is also recommended when a patient or surrogate makes treatment decisions about life-sustaining and emergency interventions. This process should anticipate the possibility that emergency medical personnel may be summoned to a home in response to an emergency call concerning an individual with documented treatment preferences, and that the person who placed the call may or may not be aware of these preferences. Professionals who conduct advance care planning and professionals authorized to write medical orders should confirm whether the emergency medical service in the community where a patient lives will honor out-of-hospital orders, including a DNR order in a set of portable medical orders, and ensure that the patient and the patient's caregivers know how to provide this documentation to EMS personnel. The responsible professional should also inform patients, surrogates, and others involved in a patient's care about any situation in which a documented decision about emergency treatment may not be honored and what measures patients and surrogates may be able to take to prevent this. The responsible professional should explain the possible consequences of calling 911 when a patient's condition is deteriorating.

On occasion, a patient with a standing DNR order may wish to receive a treatment, such as a surgical procedure, raising the question of whether the DNR order should be temporarily suspended or modified so the patient can receive the desired treatment, or whether the order should be maintained during the delivery of the treatment. Professionals responsible for the ongoing medical care of patients with DNR orders and other professionals who may become involved in the care of these patients to deliver specific treatments should know the status of all standing medical orders. They should address with the patient or surrogate how a desired and medically appropriate treatment (such as surgery) may affect a standing order, and they should describe all options for proceeding so the patient or surrogate can make an informed choice. In the event that a standing order is temporarily suspended or modified, this should be carefully documented.

For additional guidance on decisions about CPR and DNR orders, see Part Three, Section 4D.

**Nurses and other team members should alert the responsible professional if documented orders do not address the situation at hand. The responsible professional should promptly respond to the need for new orders.**

Nurses comprise the single largest health care profession in the United States. Licensed registered nurses (RNs) have immense responsibility for the hands-on delivery of end-of-life care in all care settings. Advanced practice registered nurses (APRNs), also known as nurse practitioners, have additional academic and clinical training and are certified as specialists. Nurse Practice Acts in each state define the roles and authority of different types of nurses. Activities that fall within the nursing "scope of practice" can be initiated by a registered nurse. Other activities require a registered nurse to collaborate with a physician. Nurses should know the law of the state in which they practice, including law relevant to their care settings or specialties and to activities such as prescribing medications.

Bedside nurses frequently rely on documentation originating with other health care professionals to provide round-the-clock medical and nursing care to seriously ill patients. Documents used by registered nurses and by some other team members include orders written by physicians, nurse-practitioners, or physician assistants following treatment decisions by patients or surrogates. Orders communicate treatment decisions to members of the health care team. A patient's decision about CPR or another life-sustaining treatment that was made prior to hospitalization and is reflected in an advance directive should also be documented to guide inpatient care.

Bedside care is impeded when documentation does not address the situation at hand. For example, when a loved one perceives that a hospitalized patient is in distress due to pain and changing the current pain management plan requires a new order, the patient may suffer while the bedside professional awaits the necessary authorization, if this professional cannot issue a new order.

To prevent suffering and reduce disruptions in patient care, all professionals with authority to write orders should recognize that another team member may need swift clarification or updating of orders documenting treatment decisions or care preferences. This team member is often a nurse because of the central role this professional plays in patient care. Nursing homes, hospice programs, and home care agencies should clarify how nurses and physicians can collaborate to write and revise orders when physicians may not be closely involved in day-to-day care. Academic medical centers, where early-career house staff (interns, resident physicians, and fellows) are often responsible for a patient's care, should also consider how to support this aspect of professional collaboration.

For related guidance on continuity of care across shift changes and care settings, see Part Two, Section 4.

In the interest of continuity of care, institutional policies and procedures should ensure that adequate records, including documentation of treatment decisions, travel with patients across care settings. These *Guidelines* recommend the use of portable medical orders.

Communication among professionals and paraprofessionals caring for the same patient across different care settings is difficult. Miscommunications or poorly coordinated logistics during transfer or discharge lead to breakdowns in the continuity of care and the increased likelihood that a patient's treatment decisions and care plan will not be honored. When patients are being transferred to different institutions or discharged to hospice or home care, the institution that has been caring for the patient has an obligation to develop a discharge plan that will ensure continuity of care and that the patient's or surrogate's treatment decisions will work in the new setting. This requires full documentation and communication of advance directives, treatment decisions, and standing orders. As different institutions vary in their use of advance care planning and their documentation policies and procedures, a set of portable medical orders will help to ensure patient well-being by clarifying previous treatment decisions. For additional guidance on care transitions, see Part Two, Section 4.

## G. Implementing the Decision

If a time-limited trial is consistent with a patient's goals of care, it is ethically preferable to offer a time-limited trial of a treatment that has potential for benefit and to withdraw it if it fails, rather than to rule it out without offering a trial. The patient or surrogate may refuse a time-limited trial.

In a time-limited trial, an intervention is started with the prior understanding that after a defined period, the desirability of continuing the treatment will be reassessed. Time-limited trials will not be possible for all treatments. However, when a time-limited trial is possible, the responsible professional should offer this option, with evaluation after an agreed-upon time, for any life-sustaining treatment a patient or surrogate is considering starting or continuing. A trial period can help assess the benefits and burdens of a treatment if these are difficult to assess in advance. A trial period may also reduce a patient's fears of losing the ability to stop treatment after making a decision to start it or help a patient or loved ones to be at peace with a subsequent decision to withdraw treatment.

The responsible professional should explain all burdens associated with any proposed time-limited trial. If the patient's overall condition is irreversibly deteriorating, burdensome interventions should not be attempted or continued.

The care of patients who may be in the last days and hours of life, and of these patients' loved ones, requires clear communication about the expected stages of the dying process and continuous access to palliative care.

Patients, surrogates, and loved ones may find the aftermath of a decision to forgo treatment stressful if they have not been prepared for the signs and symptoms of the dying process. Ongoing support from members of the health care team who can explain what is happening to the patient and provide comfort and reassurance is part of good palliative care at the end of life. For additional guidance concerning the care of the dying patient and of loved ones, see Part Three, Sections 3 and 4.

## H. Changing Treatment Decisions

Patients with decision-making capacity are entitled to revisit and change a treatment decision. Surrogate decision-makers can also revisit and change a treatment decision applying surrogate decision-making standards.

Patients with decision-making capacity can change their decision concerning a life-sustaining treatment at any time. Following the standards for surrogate decision-making described above (see Part Two, Section 2D, "Surrogate Decision-Making"), the surrogate for a patient without decision-making capacity can also at any time change a decision concerning a life-sustaining treatment, provided that the change is consistent with the patient's explicit preferences; or, in the absence of these, the patient's inferred values and preferences; or, if these cannot be known, the patient's best interests. The responsible professional should always be prepared to discuss the possibility of changing a decision with the patient or surrogate. Any change and the reasons for it should be documented in the patient's records.

If a patient or loved ones discuss new treatment preferences or a desire to revisit a treatment decision during informal conversations with members of the health care team, the team member with this new information should alert the responsible professional.

Every team member shares responsibility for relaying new information relevant to decision-making to the professional responsible for directing a patient's care. Simply noting these conversations in the patient's health records does not ensure that the responsible professional will see and follow up on the note. The responsible professional should be receptive to new information and should be prepared to follow up with the patient or surrogate.

## I. Conflicts and Challenges Related to Treatment Decision-Making

The responsible professional should know how to recognize and manage conflicts that may arise during treatment decision-making. Institutions should offer resources to professionals on how to address conflicts.

Health care team members should know the common sources of conflicts in making decisions about life-sustaining treatment and in care near the end of life. They should know how to act to prevent conflicts when possible and how to resolve conflicts when they cannot be prevented. Even when a patient's preferences have been documented, conflicts about treatment decision-making can arise due to poor communication, inconclusive clinical information, disagreements among loved ones, or unresolved tension within the health care team. Institutional processes should include processes for managing conflict, such as processes for addressing challenges to determinations concerning a patient's decision-making capacity or a surrogate's decision-making authority. These processes include ethics consultation.

For example, the surrogate for a patient who lacks decision-making capacity may express the personal belief that life in the patient's current condition is "not worth living." However, the patient may have expressed different values and preferences. The responsible professional and other team members should remind the surrogate to follow the patient's values and preferences when these are known. If the responsible professional has concerns about the ability of this surrogate to make treatment decisions in keeping with the standards for surrogate decision-making (see Part Two, Section 2D, "Surrogate Decision-Making," above), the professional may seek an ethics consultation to determine whether the surrogate understands the obligations of surrogate decision-making and can discharge them. On occasion, judicial review may be necessary.

**A patient who has been determined to lack decision-making capacity should be able to challenge both that determination and a surrogate's decision.**

Determining that a patient lacks decision-making capacity has grave consequences for the patient. It means that the patient is no longer functioning as the primary decision-maker. Yet the patient still has the greatest stake in decisions about his or her treatment. The patient must be able to challenge the determination that he or she lacks decision-making capacity, and also to challenge a surrogate's decision. The challenge should be referred to the ethics consultation service, ethics committee, or other institutional mechanism for prompt review. Judicial review may also be necessary.

**When a member of the health care team is concerned that a patient's ability to make decisions is impaired due to undue pressure from loved ones or other persons, the team member should promptly contact the responsible professional so the professional can determine the patient's current wishes and preferences.**

The responsible professional should interview the patient privately to determine whether the patient expresses different preferences when others are not present. The responsible professional may wish to involve other professionals, from mental health, social work, or chaplaincy, in the patient interview, or to call for an ethics consultation to get help in determining whether the patient's decision is being made under undue pressure. The responsible professional should be available to support the patient when the patient's decision is explained to loved ones or others involved in the patient's care. Team members should be mindful that a patient's decision-making can be influenced by the patient's personal relationships and affiliations without necessarily constituting undue pressure, and that any patient with decision-making capacity may choose to consult with loved ones or others.

**Any team member should be able to discuss ethical concerns with the responsible professional.**

Physicians, nurses, and other professionals on the health care team each have their own ethical obligations to patients. A team member with ethical concerns about treatment decision-making or patient care should bring these concerns to the responsible professional to consider. Institutions should seek to prevent the escalation of disagreements by establishing effective, nonpunitive processes for team members from different professions and specialties to air differing perspectives, resolve disagreements, and determine whether they require an ethics consultation on patient care. However, a practice of using ethics consultations to avoid resolving everyday disagreements should not be encouraged. For guidance on resolving clinical disagreements prior to decision-making discussions, see Part Three, Section 1.

**Health care professionals asserting a conscientious objection must continue to fulfill their duty of care, which requires health care professionals and institutions not to abandon their patients or interfere with patients' access to care by others. Health care professionals have an obligation to inform their superiors and fellow team members about any treatment options they find morally objectionable well in advance of any situation in which a conflict may arise.**

If a health care professional objects to implementing the treatment decision of a patient or surrogate on religious or other moral grounds, the professional may assert a conscientious objection to participating and may seek to withdraw from the case. However, a conscientious objection should rest on a basic moral commitment or principle that the professional can articulate. It is inappropriate to assert a conscientious objection simply because the professional prefers a different treatment decision or would make a different treatment decision in his or her own care. The health care professional has an obligation to notify the patient or surrogate of this objection as early as possible and to protect patient well-being by assisting in the orderly and prompt transfer of the patient to a professional who can act in keeping with the patient's or surrogate's treatment decision. Informing superiors and team members about conscientious objections in advance may help in accommodating the objection without interfering with patient care. If transferring a case is impossible because of the patient's condition or because no other professional will accept the patient, the responsible professional should follow the patient's or surrogate's treatment choices and may request an ethics consultation.

For guidance on conscientious objection by health care institutions with formal religious commitments, see Part Two, Section 6G.

For additional guidance on the role of ethics consultation and conflict resolution in addressing conflict and challenges related to treatment decision-making, see Part Two, Section 6A and 6G.

# Guidelines Concerning Neonates, Infants, Children, and Adolescents

## Introduction

The ethical and legal framework that informs these *Guidelines* also supports treatment decision-making involving minors. This section discusses the additional special considerations that arise when discussions and decision-making occur in pediatric care settings and involve the medical treatment of minors of different ages and developmental stages.[19] Professionals who work in pediatric care settings or in institutions that provide care to minors and adults are encouraged to use this section in the context of the full document, as other sections include material that can support good care for pediatric patients and their loved ones.

Approximately 50,000 deaths occur among pediatric patients in the United States each year, and more than half of these occur during the first year of life.[20] Many of these deaths in infancy are the result of extreme prematurity and marginal viability. The neonatal and pediatric intensive care units (NICU and PICU, respectively) are the most common settings for decision-making about pediatric life-sustaining treatment.

Children and adolescents may die from a range of causes, including life-threatening health problems resulting from congenital abnormalities or rare inherited disorders, or from cancer, other acute disease, or trauma. Many children and adolescents die in hospitals, although policy reforms at the state level are gradually increasing pediatric services available through hospice programs and home care programs. Some children and adolescents live in residential long-term care facilities and may die in these settings.

Pediatric decision-making is a special form of surrogate decision-making that usually involves both the child (if old enough to understand treatment choices) and the parent or guardian. Both law and ethics recognize that as children grow in their capacity to understand and participate in decisions about their medical care, their role in decision-making should also grow. Indeed, some older adolescents may have decision-making capacity and so may be able to decide for themselves. This category includes adolescents who are making medical decisions as mature minors or as emancipated minors as recognized by statute or case law. The standards for surrogate decision-making described in Part Two, Section 2, are discussed below with reference to different pediatric contexts. The guidelines for determining decision-making capacity—also in Part Two, Section 2—should be consulted when conducting a clinical evaluation of an older adolescent whose decision-making capacity has not been established.

These *Guidelines* refer to children from one through six years of age as "young children" and to those from *approximately* seven years of age (as decision-making capacity begins to develop) through *approximately* thirteen years of age as "older children." "Adolescents" refers to those from *approximately* fourteen through seventeen years of age, with those nearing adulthood referred to as "older adolescents." These age ranges roughly represent developmental stages, not hard categories.

By law, persons who are eighteen years of age or older are adults, not children. Some adults may receive medical care in pediatric settings to maintain continuity of care following a childhood diagnosis, and some insurers may continue to cover legal adults up to a certain age as dependent children or as persons eligible for coverage as pediatric patients. With respect to treatment decision-making, the *Guidelines* for adult patients apply to all adults receiving care, even if in pediatric settings, and through any insurance mechanism.

## Treatment decision-making as part of family-centered care

The philosophy of care in pediatric settings tends to be "family-centered" (or "family-focused"), reflecting the broad professional consensus in pediatric medicine that patients who are children are likely to be accompanied and supported by parents or guardians, and that caring for a child also requires caring for the child's loved ones and being attentive to the impact of a child's illness and treatment on relationships within a family. Offering parents or guardians places to sleep and shower while remaining close to the child's bedside and offering child care for well siblings during hospital visits are some tangible examples of family-centered care.

Treatment decision-making for children should respect their family context. In health care as in other aspects of their lives, children are neither developmentally nor legally equivalent to autonomous adults. However, surrogate decision-making standards designed with incapacitated adults in mind are not a precise fit for the situation of children and adolescents. By law, children cannot execute legally binding advance directives, although portable medical orders reflecting patient preferences may be authorized for use in the care of pediatric patients in some states. The expressed preference and substituted judgment standards, in which a surrogate decision-maker is guided by the patient's explicit preferences if known or by the patient's inferred values and preferences, are problematic to follow before a young child has had an opportunity to form and communicate preferences that can guide a surrogate. However, by the age of seven, a developmentally typical child may be capable of assenting to (or dissenting from) a surrogate's decision. By fourteen years of age, adolescents may be capable of making informed choices about many aspects of their lives, including medical treatment. In some areas of medical decision-making, state law may explicitly recognize adolescents' independent authority at this point. Health care professionals working in pediatric settings should know the laws of the state in which they practice.

Children vary in their capacity for involvement in treatment decision-making. Some younger children have levels of maturity equivalent to that of an adolescent with respect to their ability to understand and reflect on their condition and its treatment. A child diagnosed early in life may also have more experience as a patient than does a newly diagnosed adolescent.

Current professional guidance in pediatric and adolescent medicine reflects extensive research and consensus-building concerning the ability of children and younger adolescents to participate in medical decision-making and the ability of older adolescents to make informed decisions. The Bibliography supporting this section includes a selection of empirical literature and professional recommendations on these topics. The web-based research and educational resources included in the Bibliography offer additional material on pediatric decision-making and care.

## Best interests decision-making for children

When a patient is an infant or a young child, or is older but is unable to express preferences or to indicate their values and participate in decision-making, the best interests standard provides the framework for discussing and making an ethical decision. As described in Part Two, Section 2D, "(Surrogate Decision-Making)," this is because the patient does not have decision-making capacity and the patient's explicit preferences and values relevant to the decision at hand cannot reliably be inferred. The application of the best interests standard involves considering factors such as the patient's apparent experience of his or her illness or condition; whether the patient appears to be suffering physically or psychologically; the treatment options with some realistic potential for benefiting this patient; the benefits and burdens of each of these treatment options, including the option to forgo further life-sustaining interventions; and the patient's ability to understand and tolerate the treatment. The best interests standard should be applied in a way that is tailored to the clinical circumstances and particular experiences of this child with reference to current clinical facts, treatment options, and the patient's present and predicted experience and quality of life. For example, the discussion of what most but not all patients of this child's age and developmental stage would experience as treatment "benefits" or treatment "burdens" should take into account this child's particular interests and also the experiential and/or developmental consequences of different treatment options for this still-developing child. This is discussed further below and in the general guidelines that follow (see Part Two, Section 3A, "General Guidelines for Pediatric Decision-Making Concerning the Use of Life-Sustaining Treatments," below).

The best interests standard does not require the continuation of efforts to sustain life in all cases. Initiating or continuing treatment that is inconsistent with the goals of care for a patient would be incompatible with this standard. A proposed treatment may also be too burdensome for the child, or its potential benefits too remote. Moreover, as discussed in Part Two, Section 2, offering or continuing treatment that cannot provide physiological benefit with the goal of potentially offering some psychological benefit is ethically problematic for several reasons. It adds burden for the patient, no matter what psychological effect it may offer for the patient or for parents or guardians. It may involve a form of deception, through "pretending" that a treatment has potential for physiological benefit when it does not. Finally, it fails to address directly the underlying psychological needs. The responsible professional should seek to address the patient's psychological needs and those of parents or guardians directly, through mental health services and through professional collaboration with palliative care and hospice specialists.

## Assent, dissent, and parental permission in decision-making with pediatric patients

As noted, children who are at least seven years old and are capable of participating in treatment decision-making are capable of agreeing to a surrogate's decision (*assent*) or disagreeing with this decision (*dissent*). Federal guidelines on human subjects research generally require the *assent* of participants who are younger than eighteen and capable of providing assent, plus informed *permission* from parents or guardians.[21] Assent and dissent in treatment decision-making with children and the participation of adolescents in decision-making are discussed in greater detail in the guidelines that follow.

## Collaboration in pediatric decision-making

Professionals responsible for the care of pediatric patients should be prepared to support the involvement of children and adolescents, as well as parents or guardians, in decision-making. Health care professionals should also know how treatment decision-making may unfold in different pediatric care settings. Deliberation about potential treatment decisions may begin before birth, when the birth of a severely ill or imperiled newborn is expected. Parents or guardians may need support to make health care decisions for their child. The rarity of some life-threatening conditions affecting children means that parents or guardians may not know anyone who has faced the particular decisions they face. Health care professionals may also have less experience caring for pediatric patients with extremely rare conditions and, therefore, less experience supporting decision-makers under those circumstances.

Family-centered care settings should anticipate that treatment decision-making will involve parents or guardians, the patient (as able), and health care professionals, including physicians, nurses, child-life specialists, social workers, chaplains, and others; such settings should promote ongoing collaboration among these individuals. A collaborative approach can both support decision-makers and also provide a reliable structure for information-sharing and discussions. For example, in some cases a primary nurse who is assigned to the patient and provides bedside care whenever he or she is on duty provides continuity of care for the patient and family. Institutions should offer ethics education to health care professionals working in pediatric settings to support their collaboration with parents or guardians as soon as a child is diagnosed with a progressive or life-threatening condition and the family begins to cope with the child's condition. The Bibliography includes resources on collaboration in pediatric care. For additional discussion of communication relevant to treatment decision-making, see Part Three.

## The pediatric patient's perspective in decision-making

Helping the sick child to bring his or her own voice and perspective into treatment decision-making is an ethical obligation and a practical challenge. Children express themselves differently than do adults. They may know much more about their diagnosis, prognosis, and treatment than adults realize. Even a young child may be aware that he or she is very sick and dying. Individual children differ in what they care about and what they wish to avoid. A child whose diet is severely restricted may still value the social ritual of going out for ice cream with friends or grandparents. An adolescent may want to know if he can still go swimming if he opts to get a port implanted for intravenous medication, and what the port will look and feel like. These patients and their parents or guardians may need health care professionals to reassure them that these preferences matter.

Some of these preferences and concerns may be developmentally typical and predictable. For example, an adolescent tends to be more concerned than a preadolescent about outward appearance and peer attitudes. This may mean that an adolescent may be more concerned than a younger child about treatment consequences that would temporarily affect his or her appearance or disrupt peer relationships. A child who loves school may be particularly concerned about missing school due to treatment. Discussions with children about treatment decision-making should take these concerns seriously by addressing the disruptions that treatment may bring to the life of the patient, how the patient feels about these potential disruptions, and how these disruptions can be minimized. Electronic decision-making tools have been developed for use in pediatric settings; these tools may engage some children and adolescents, provide them with information about treatment, and help to elicit their preferences.

What a child likes to do is a huge part of who a child is. Discussions of treatment options should aim to include the child's perspective on how he or she likes to spend time right now to help decision-makers assess the benefits and burdens of treatment as they will be experienced by this still-developing person. The values of family-centered care should not slip into treating the parent or guardian as the patient, a notion that obscures the identity of the patient and may undermine the patient's own role in decision-making. Eliciting the preferences of children who may not be able to readily articulate their preferences may take time and involve different members of the health care team ranging from child-life specialists and art therapists to pediatric chaplains and pediatric social workers.

One question for patients or guardians that can start a process of collaboration that is family-centered is "Who is your child?" By inviting parents or guardians—and the child, as he or she is able—to talk about who the child is as a person, as a family member, and as a community member, health care professionals convey their respect for the child as a person and for the child's relationships. This demonstration of early and sincere interest in the child's identity, interests, and relationships may serve as a touchstone in difficult days ahead.

## A. General Guidelines for Pediatric Decision-Making Concerning the Use of Life-Sustaining Treatments

Pediatric care settings should support those involved in decision-making, provide a reliable structure for information-sharing and for discussions about treatment decisions, and train staff to communicate and collaborate effectively with patients and parents or guardians in the decision-making process.

An ethically sound approach to collaboration in pediatric care settings should include:

### Shared information

All participants in decision-making discussions—including all professionals who may be responsible for a child's care or who may take part in family conferences—should understand the goals of the discussion and be provided with current medical and other information relevant to the discussion. This includes the child or adolescent who is participating in any way in the decision-making process. The presentation to the patient should be appropriate to his or her level of comprehension. Professionals should aim to describe the process of treatment decision-making in advance so those involved in decision-making know what to expect as different decisions need to be made.

### Medical conference prior to family conference

The objective of the medical conference is to elicit clinical perspectives relevant to the needs of the whole child, rather than focusing on problems in isolation, and to identify any disagreements within the team. Communicating and reconciling specialist recommendations in advance of the family conference sets the stage for good decision-making. If the family conference will take place in a hospital, the medical conference should also aim to include clinical perspectives from the patient's out-of-hospital team, which may include hospice providers if the patient is receiving concurrent hospice care, and also primary care providers and home care providers.

### Patient involvement in the family conference

Whenever the patient is able to play a role in the decision-making, he or she should be included in any family conference at which decision-making is expected to occur. There may be a need for additional conferences to support the family as they cope with the patient's condition and their own stress.

### Time and place for family conferences

Professionals should allow ample time for family conferences that will include discussion and decision-making about life-sustaining treatment. A conference room or other quiet, private space should be available to professionals, the patient (when involved in decision-making), and family. Sometimes the patient's condition will require that the conference be held at the patient's bedside. Medical emergencies may on occasion limit the time and privacy available for family conferences.

### Continuity

Families and patients themselves may feel burdened if they have to present the patient's medical history alone and repeatedly. At least one professional who is knowledgeable about the child's history and care should participate in each family conference to provide support as needed. Depending on the needs of the patient and family, this help may be provided by a case manager, a palliative care specialist, a social worker, or the nurse with primary responsibility for bedside care.

### Goals of care

Once the goals of care have been established with the patient (if able) and parents or guardians, all subsequent discussions about pending or potential treatment decisions should address new information about the patient's condition or the burdens or benefits of treatment options with reference to the established goals. This promotes continuity of care as well as ethical outcomes.

### Discussion and decision-making

When professionals, patients, and families have already established a collaborative relationship, they may be able to discuss treatment options, the patient's values and preferences (if they are known or can be inferred) and best interests, and any clinical recommendations to reach a decision during the family conference. Some patients and families may need additional time for reflection or the opportunity to talk with clinical experts or trusted individuals before a decision can be reached. If the child is able to provide information about his or her values and preferences or will be playing a larger decision-making role by offering assent, dissent, or consent, it will be necessary to allow time to elicit the child's views, either as part of the family conference or in addition to it.

## Identification of needs resulting from decision

The collaborative process should identify what the patient and family may need as the result of a particular decision. For example, a decision to forgo further life-sustaining interventions should include a plan for meeting the palliative care needs of the patient, including any new needs as a result of the treatment decision, and a plan for providing support to the family for the remainder of the child's life. A decision involving a care transition should include a palliative care plan that can be sustained in the new care setting and close attention to care coordination as the patient's care is transferred to a different unit or institution or to the family. (See Part Two, Section 4.) A decision to begin a time-limited trial should provide for communication among professionals, the patient, and the family as the treatment's desirability is assessed.

## Documentation and implementation

The decision-making process should include documentation of treatment goals and treatment decisions, as well as the implementation of these decisions. It is important to document the relative roles of the patient and parents or guardians in the decision-making process so that future decision-making continues to respect those roles; if the child or adolescent is already providing assent, dissent, or consent, that role needs to be respected as decision-making progresses. This documentation should be integrated into the patient's medical record so it is available across shifts and care settings.

Ethical processes for decision-making about life-sustaining treatments and the goals of care should explicitly clarify what role the child or adolescent will play, including whether the child or adolescent will be asked for assent, dissent, or consent.

If an older adolescent is being asked to give informed consent, the decision-making process should aim to elicit the patient's preferences. In all other cases, the decision-making process should aim to identify the patient's preferences and values or infer them based on knowledge of and experience with the patient, identify the parents' or guardians' view of those preferences and values, and clarify parents' or guardians' perceptions of a child's best interests. The involvement of professionals with expertise in communication can support this process.

Treatment decision-making for children or adolescents can be complex. It may not be clear to all involved—including the patient and parents or guardians—what the decision-making role of the child or adolescent is. Clarifying this is essential to an ethical decision-making process. Such clarification also allows the patient and parents or guardians to raise questions and object if they disagree with the responsible professional's expectation of the patient's decision-making role. This allows direct discussion of this important issue. Ethics consultation may be needed. Once the decision-making role of the child or adolescent is clarified, decision-making can proceed based on that shared understanding.

If an older adolescent is being asked to give informed consent, eliciting the patient's own treatment preferences is key. If the patient is not an older adolescent, the patient (if able) and the parents or guardians will both have major roles in decision-making. In either case, establishing a collaborative process involves sharing both medical information and information about values and preferences, as well as best interests. The professional with current responsibility for the patient's care is likely to have access to the medical information immediately relevant to the decision at hand. However, the pediatric patient's full medical history may be better known to the patient and parents or guardians than to the current treating physician, depending on where and how long the patient has been receiving treatment. The patient and parents or guardians are the key sources of information about values and preferences relevant to the decision. Parents or guardians are also the key judges of their child's best interests.

Professionals should be aware that they often bring their own values into the discussion, especially if asked, "If this were your child, what would you do?" A professional's clinical recommendation should be based on the professional's assessment of the current medical facts and what the professional has heard from the child and parents or guardians concerning the child's values and preferences (if those are explicit or can be inferred) and best interests. It is preferable to offer a clinical recommendation in a way that is compassionate and that acknowledges that the professional is not the parent ("As your child's physician…"). To present a clinical recommendation in terms of the professional's own values ("If this were my child…") may be problematic, as it may obscure the preferences of the patient and the judgment of the parents or guardians. Also, some parents or guardians may be distressed by the suggestion that a professional is able to imagine what their personal experience of their child's illness and treatment is like.

Professionals such as social workers, chaplains, child-life specialists and other mental health professionals, palliative care specialists, and nurse managers can support collaboration. They may act as facilitators during family conferences or be available for support during and after decision-making. Offering parents or guardians opportunities to talk with other family caregivers who can provide perspectives on the possible long-term consequences of a treatment decision can also be helpful.

## Family-centered care in different pediatric care settings should be organized to support effective collaboration in decision-making in each of these settings.

Parents or guardians of a critically ill infant or a child newly diagnosed with a life-threatening disease face challenges that differ from those faced by parents or guardians with years of experience caring for a child or adolescent with a chronic or recurrent condition. The collaborative process used in intensive-care settings is also likely to differ from a process used in chronic-care settings, while a process used in a perinatal-care setting or NICU will differ from a process in which an older child is able to participate.

As collaboration requires communication, sustaining an ethically sound process for treatment decision-making in pediatric care contexts requires attention to competence in communication. Ethics education in institutions that provide pediatric care should support this aspect of practice by offering regular opportunities for pediatric care professionals, including resident physicians and other early-career professionals, to improve their communication skills. For additional guidance, see Part One, Section 2, and Part Three.

**Parents or guardians should be supported so they are not overwhelmed by the burden of responsibility for decisions concerning a child's life-sustaining treatment.**

Parents and guardians may not want to feel alone in decisions about a child's care, especially in the case of young children unable to play a significant role in treatment decision-making. It may be overwhelming to feel they hold life-or-death power in this circumstance or that the child could suffer as a consequence of their decision. They may need reassurance that their decision makes sense. Within a collaborative process, it is ethically appropriate for professionals to ease the burden of such decisions. Presenting treatment options with reference to established goals of care and clearly explaining how various options now under consideration reflect these goals can support decision-makers.

If a decision to continue life-sustaining treatment may result in a severe impairment due to the child's underlying condition or as a consequence of treatment, the responsible professional should provide parents or guardians with accurate information about this impairment and its consequences for the child's development, including the ability to pursue activities known to be of interest to this child or to children of this child's age. For example, radiation to treat brain tumors in infants and young children can affect a child's development and neurocognition, with the potential for severe impairment in some cases. Extremely premature infants who require extensive use of a ventilator in the first weeks or months of life may develop chronic and potentially serious lung problems. Offering parents or guardians the opportunity to talk with a professional or a family caregiver with expert knowledge of the long-term experience and consequences of a particular impairment is helpful, as the responsible professional may not possess this expert knowledge. Palliative care consultation may also help parents or guardians to learn about the palliative care needs that may be associated with a particular impairment and how these needs would be met.

Whenever a decision to forgo treatment is likely to result in death, the collaborative decision-making process should include a palliative care specialist or other professional who can address end-of-life care in the setting in which death is likely to occur, with attention to support for the child through the dying process and family bereavement. Eliciting a child's own preferences about where and how to spend the rest of his or her life is of immense importance. What a dying child is interested in may be the soundest guide to good care at the end of life.

**When collaborative deliberations reveal but fail to resolve a conflict over decision-making between the patient and others or between a family and the health care team, the responsible professional should request an ethics consultation or other**

conflict resolution intervention. The patient, as well as parents or guardians and other team members, should be able to request these services.

Conflicts that may require ethics consultation or third-party conflict resolution may arise from disagreements between the child and parents or guardians, between parents or guardians, or between any of these individuals and members of the health care team. In the interest of preventing harm due to delays in decision-making or the continuation of treatment that is burdening but not benefiting the patient, these conflicts must be addressed promptly.

Occasionally, conflicts arise within the health care team itself. Family-centered care should be designed to prevent decision-making conflicts that arise from poorly coordinated care or from unresolved professional tensions. For example, staff members who disagree with a colleague's treatment recommendation or the implementation of a surrogate's decision to continue life-sustaining treatment may feel distressed or angry if, *in their perception*, adults are "allowing a child to suffer." On the other hand, distress and anger among staff may also be triggered by the *perception* that a child is being denied life-sustaining treatment and "not being given a chance." Parents or guardians who become aware of these perceptions and emotions may in turn become distressed or angry. The potential for communication problems and unresolved distress to undermine collaboration in pediatric settings should be recognized and addressed by institutions through ethics education and conflict resolution. For additional guidance, see Part Two, Section 6, and Part Three, Section 3G ("Moral Distress as a Factor in Treatment Decision-Making").

## When it is unclear who exercises surrogate decision-making authority on behalf of a child, ethics consultation is needed.

Decisions concerning children in the foster care system should be made with reference to guidance clarifying who can make medical decisions involving a child for whom the state has custody. Institutions may provide this guidance in the form of a written procedure on how decision-making should proceed in these cases in light of state law. If procedural guidance is not available or does not address the situation at hand, ethics consultation is necessary.

Situations in which the responsible professional has concerns about the ability of parents or guardians to discharge the responsibilities of surrogate decision-makers or in which responsibility for surrogate decision-making is unclear for some other reason should also include ethics consultation. Consultation with legal counsel and legal proceedings to clarify decision-making authority may be required as well.

Education in institutions that care for pediatric patients should cover law, regulations, and institutional policy relevant to decision-making by parents or guardians and the rights of minors themselves. Education should prepare responsible professionals to work with these standards in collaborative decision-making and to suggest when to seek guidance from ethics consultation or institutional legal counsel. For additional material on the role of ethics services in supporting treatment decision-making, see Part Two, Section 6A

("Guidelines on Ethics Services in Institutions Providing Care for Patients Facing Decisions about Life-Sustaining Treatment or Approaching the End of Life").

**Palliative care for children is ethically obligatory. It should be integrated into all health care settings that provide care to pediatric patients with chronic, progressive, or life-threatening conditions.**

Children need and deserve relief from suffering. Pediatric health care professionals have an obligation to act to prevent and relieve suffering. Interdisciplinary pediatric palliative care is grounded in this fundamental moral principle and aims to respond to pain, symptoms, and suffering resulting from a child's illness and its treatment. As the diagnosis and treatment of a life-threatening illness in a child is also likely to affect that child's entire family, pediatric palliative care is essential in family-centered care. Pain and symptom management should be integrated into all treatment plans for neonates, infants, children, and adolescents. Access to supportive services, such as mental health care, child-life care, chaplaincy, and social work, should be integrated into all treatment plans for pediatric patients. Children's hospitals should have pediatric palliative care teams. Institutions that care for both adults and children should include specialists in pediatric palliative care on their palliative care teams or should create a specialized pediatric palliative care team. Patients with chronic disease may need palliative care services that are accessible across care settings, including the home.

Children's hospitals, as well as institutions that include pediatric subpopulations, should collect data on palliative care needs associated with different diagnoses. Using these data to identify unmet needs with the goal of improving access to palliative care for pediatric patients throughout an institution can reduce professional uncertainty about how to integrate palliative care into medical treatment effectively and how to collaborate with palliative care specialists.

**Hospice care is an ethically appropriate option for patients who are children.**

As these *Guidelines* have discussed, treatment plans that are not aimed at prolonging a child's life are ethically acceptable. A terminally ill child may have much to lose if he or she is burdened by treatment with small potential for benefit, rather than spending his or her remaining time in ways that are likely to be more comforting and satisfying. A belief that this child has "nothing left to lose," if treatment continues until death, fails to consider the value of this child's remaining time and the child's own preferences.

Without explicit discussion, it may be difficult for parents or guardians to imagine what opting to forgo further efforts to prolong a child's life would look like, including such basic questions as where the child would live out his or her remaining life, how pain and symptoms would be managed and supportive services delivered outside of an inpatient setting, and how they would simultaneously care for a dying child and the child's siblings. Responsibility for discussing and coordinating hospice-level palliative care, whether or not a child is formally enrolled in hospice, is likely to fall to hospital-based professionals responsible for a child's care. As access to hospice care for children who are still receiving therapeutic treatment is expanding through the state-level implementation of the "concurrent care for children" provision of the Patient Protection and Affordable Care Act of 2010 (see Part One, Section 4B, "Economic Context"), professionals should be prepared to discuss local hospice services that may be available to children while they are receiving treatment.

In situations where forgoing further efforts to prolong life may be in keeping with the child's values and preferences (if they are known or can be inferred) and best interests, the responsible professional, or a palliative care professional with expertise in pediatric care, should discuss with parents or guardians the option to forgo further life-sustaining interventions and continue palliative care for the rest of the child's life. Palliative care team members in institutions that provide care to pediatric patients should be familiar with available pediatric hospice programs and able to discuss these services with parents or guardians and with the child (if he or she is able) and to help arrange services as desired. If no pediatric hospice program is available, the pediatric palliative care team should work with the responsible professional and the parents or guardians and the child (if able) to develop a plan for palliative care that will continue through the remainder of the child's life.

## Collaborative decision-making should promote continuity of care within and across pediatric care settings.

Responsibility for coordinating the care of a pediatric patient often falls to a parent or guardian. Family-centered care should encompass care coordination that allows family caregivers to share this responsibility, if they choose, with a professional. Offering families access to a care coordinator who can assist with care transitions within and across care settings is recommended. Pediatric care settings that do not offer professional care coordination should, at minimum, acknowledge the burdens of parents or guardians who bear sole responsibility for care coordination. Family-centered care should aim to minimize this burden through a collaborative decision-making process in which all professionals participate that offers a structure for identifying care-coordination needs, and through the involvement of palliative care specialists in transfers and discharge planning. For additional guidance on care transitions, see Part Two, Section 4.

## B. Guidelines for Decision-Making and Care Involving Nonviable Neonates and Neonates at the Threshold of Viability

In cases where a pregnant woman is at high risk for delivering an extremely premature neonate, perinatal care should include preparation for the prospect of best interest decision-making for the child in the NICU following the delivery.

Perinatologists or other specialists involved in the care of pregnant women at high risk of extremely premature delivery should initiate discussions with these patients about the treatment decisions that may arise and the potential consequences of these decisions.

These discussions—which may also involve other professionals who can provide support to the pregnant woman and to other family members—help to establish a collaborative decision-making process if the infant is born at the margins of viability.

**In cases where a nonviable neonate cannot benefit from resuscitation and stabilization attempts, comfort care should be provided until death.**

Discussions with women at high risk of extremely premature delivery should clarify the threshold of viability for a neonate, as attempting interventions that have no potential for physiological benefit would produce only pain and suffering for the child. Once the child is born and his or her nonviable condition has been confirmed, the responsible professional should describe options for palliative care and support the parents' or guardians' decision-making based on the child's best interests. Palliative care for these children, including bereavement care for their parents or guardians while the infant is dying and following death, should be provided in the delivery room or in a quiet, private space. Sometimes this space is in the NICU, even though no life-saving or life-prolonging interventions will be attempted.

**In cases where a neonate is born at the threshold of viability, professionals should describe the neonate's condition, explain resuscitation and other stabilization measures in the context of the neonate's condition, and determine the parents' decision concerning initial resuscitation and other stabilization attempts based on the best interests of the child. The extent and duration of these attempts should reflect the parents decision. If initial attempts succeed, a collaborative process should begin for subsequent treatment planning, decision-making, and family support. All interventions should be conducted as time-limited trials. Palliative care should be fully integrated into treatment.**

Neonatologists often describe neonates born at the threshold of viability as their hardest ethical cases.[22] In the United States, only 5 percent of neonates now born at twenty-two weeks gestation will survive resuscitation and stabilization following birth and will subsequently survive intensive care treatment.[23] For those who survive to discharge, the combined consequences of extreme prematurity and life-saving interventions almost always result in moderate, severe, or profound neurodevelopmental impairment. Neonates born at twenty-three to twenty-five weeks gestation are also on the current margins of viability. During these weeks, life-saving interventions have a greater potential for success, with the potential for survival to discharge increasing and the likelihood of permanent neurodevelopmental impairment decreasing with each additional week of gestational age at birth.

While decisions about the extent and duration of interventions involving extremely premature neonates tend to be framed in terms of gestational age, uncertainty over the precise date of conception and the presence of other factors relevant to viability means that it is usually not possible to determine an extremely premature neonate's prospects and an ethical course of action from estimated gestational age alone. Five factors—gestational age, birth weight, sex, antenatal exposure to steroids to aid lung development, and single or multiple birth—are relevant to whether a neonate born at the threshold of viability can tolerate rescue efforts and potentially benefit from life support until the child's lungs and other aspects of physiological development can sustain life unaided.

An extremely premature neonate whose lungs and other major organ systems (including the skin) are as yet developmentally immature is not the same as an older neonate born with a life-threatening condition that may require the temporary or permanent use of life-sustaining treatments and technologies. After a neonate is born at the threshold of viability, it may take days or weeks to determine if this neonate's condition can be stabilized so the body's systems can continue to develop. Rapid reversals and catastrophic decompensation, including brain hemorrhage, iatrogenic lung damage, and intestinal infection, may occur. Many interventions are painful.

A collaborative process for treatment decision-making by parents or guardians during the first hours, days, and possibly weeks of the life of an extremely premature neonate should reflect the general guidelines for pediatric decision-making described in Part Two, Section 3A, above. Because a neonate's condition can change so quickly, parents or guardians should know which team member is able to provide them with current information about their child's condition. The collaborative process should include frequent updates about the status of time-limited trials. This prepares parents or guardians for decisions they may need to consider and prepares team members to support best interests decision-making by parents or guardians.

The health care team for an extremely premature neonate will include neonatologists, other medical specialists, palliative care specialists, resident physicians, the primary nurse, and perhaps also a nurse-manager or other professional responsible for assisting the parents or guardians with care coordination. A chaplain, mental health specialist, or social worker may be well placed to facilitate communication among participants in collaborative decision-making while providing support to a mother who has just given birth to an extremely premature infant (or infants, if a multiple birth), and support to other family members and loved ones.

As the membership of the health care team responsible for the care of an extremely premature neonate may change frequently during the period when decisions are being discussed and made, communication within the health care team and during transfers of responsibility for patient care is integral to supporting ongoing collaboration with the patient's surrogates. The attending physician responsible for the patient's care should alert resident physicians and other team members to the importance of helping surrogates and other family members to understand the neonate's current condition and prognosis. Reporting test results or describing vital signs in isolation ("stable," "better") may undermine informed decision-making by leading parents or guardians to conclude that their child's overall health has stabilized or is improving, and to react with confusion, mistrust, or anger if the child's condition then deteriorates.

Professionals who provide care to extremely premature neonates and participate in collaborative decision-making with parents or guardians need opportunities for ethical reflection in view of the hard ethical choices presented by these treatment decisions, the particular stresses associated with this intensive-care setting, and the likelihood that early career physicians, such as resident physicians and fellows, will have significant responsibility for patient care. Institutions should support these opportunities through ethics education.

## C. Guidelines for Decision-Making about Life-Sustaining Treatment for Viable Neonates

In decision-making concerning life-sustaining treatment for a critically ill, viable newborn, the responsible professional should aim to support decision-making by parents (or other guardians) based on the best interests of the child. Ethics consultation or conflict resolution may be needed in rare cases of disagreement between parents and professionals. A rare decision to oppose the decision of parents should include ethics consultation and legal consultation and may require judicial review.

Survival rates and medical outcomes for infants born with life-threatening impairments and congenital abnormalities have improved greatly in the past two decades. Multiple life-saving and life-sustaining treatments have been developed. Conditions once inevitably fatal can sometimes now be repaired (in utero, in some cases) and impairments that once were treated as severe disabilities can now be accommodated to permit varying degrees of functioning and independent living.

Decision-making for neonates born with life-threatening conditions should be driven by the parents' or guardians' assessment of what is in the child's best interests. Distinguishing between immediate stabilization goals and the successful resolution or management of the condition may be difficult. When a condition can be resolved definitively by medical or surgical interventions following delivery, the parents or guardians will generally decide that it is in the infant's best interests to be stabilized and treated. However, the situation of this infant is not identical to that of an older patient arriving in an emergency room. The outcome of virtually any intervention involving a neonate with a life-threatening condition is uncertain, and intensive-care interventions can have long-term consequences for development. The range of treatments and technologies in the NICU can also complicate efforts to distinguish between catastrophic conditions that are incompatible with life, no matter what interventions might be attempted, and life-threatening conditions that may respond to life-sustaining treatment.

The responsible health care professional will need to help the parents or guardians understand the medical situation in order to apply the best interests standard. Making decisions about life-sustaining treatment for a neonate in such circumstances can be challenging and stressful. This may in part be due to differing perspectives about the future of an infant for whom a successful intervention at birth will result in a chronic, progressive, or recurrent life-threatening condition that may require medical and nursing care by professionals and family members. There are many such conditions, some extremely rare. Professionals should aim to offer parents or guardians opportunities to talk with professionals or family caregivers with knowledge of the particular condition and the accommodations that may be required over time. In some cases, it will be possible to offer parents or guardians the opportunity to talk with family caregivers in person. Often it will be possible to provide them with online resources, including e-mail discussion lists and informational websites designed for family caregivers. NICU professionals should themselves have opportunities to learn from fellow professionals and family caregivers with knowledge of the long-term needs and prospects of children born with life-threatening conditions. Ethics education that offers such opportunities may strengthen these professionals' ability to collaborate with parents or guardians.

**Decision-making about life-sustaining treatment in neonates and infants should be offered as time-limited trials.**

Neonatal intensive care, pediatric intensive care, and other medical and surgical care of infants born or diagnosed with life-threatening conditions involve significant prognostic uncertainty. Time-limited trials of treatment may be important to clarify benefits and burdens and thus whether to forgo or continue a treatment. However, parents or guardians should be able to refuse life-sustaining treatment without use of a time-limited trial.

## D. Guidelines for Decision-Making about Life-Sustaining Treatment for Young Children

**Decision-making for children from ages one through six should follow the best interests standard. In cases of disagreement between professionals and parents or guardians, the responsible professional should seek ethics consultation. Conflict resolution and legal consultation may be required.**

As these *Guidelines* have discussed, when a patient is younger than seven years old (or is older but unable to express or indicate preferences or participate in decision-making), the best interests standard provides the framework for discussing and making an ethical decision about medical treatment and care. This patient does not have decision-making capacity and the patient's values and preferences relevant to the decision at hand cannot reliably be known or inferred and may not yet have formed. The general guidelines for pediatric decision-making (described in Part Two, Section 3A, above) can help support best interests decision-making for young children. For detailed discussions of the best interests standard, refer to Part Two, Section 2D ("Surrogate Decision-Making") and the Introduction to Part Two, Section 3 ("Best interests decision-making for children").

## E. Guidelines for Decision-Making with Older Children

Collaborative deliberation and the decision-making process for patients of approximately seven to fourteen years of age should reflect awareness of a child's developing decision-making capacity during this stage of life. When a patient has reached the age of at least seven years and is capable of participating in treatment decision-making, the responsible professional should ascertain whether the patient assents to a surrogate's decisions.

In cases of disagreement between the patient and parents or guardians, or a decision to override the patient's dissent, the responsible professional should seek ethics consultation. Conflict resolution and legal consultation may be required.

In the treatment of older children, the child's own preferences are ethically significant. Children tend to agree with their parents or guardians on goals of care and treatment plans. However, professionals responsible for the care of children who are approximately seven to fourteen years old should be aware that older children may hold their own views. The responsible professional should ascertain whether the child assents to the decision of the parents or guardians.

Decisions about an older child's medical treatment should reflect the child's developmental maturity, including his or her values and preferences. An older child may have preferences about small but meaningful details of treatment or the health care environment—preferences that may be unknown or surprising even to parents or guardians. One child may dislike watching a nurse access a port or start an IV, while a different child (or the same child at a different age) may be fascinated by these procedures. Giving a child a choice is one way to respect this child as a person and to acknowledge the child's experience as a patient.

Treatment decision-making with older children and with their parents or guardians requires the responsible professional to understand informed assent, which assumes a collaborative decision-making process in which each participant has information and insights to contribute and in which it is acknowledged that some participants have more power and influence than others. In this process, the responsible professional should make sure that the patient's perspective is elicited, shared with other participants in the decision-making process, and remains a focal point of the discussion. The older child who participates in an informed assent process may choose to assent to the treatment decision that others endorse, or to dissent. The involvement of a pediatric mental health professional or other palliative care specialist may be helpful in eliciting the child's perspective and concerns and in building consensus. If the child dissents from the decision of the parents or guardians, ethics consultation is needed, and conflict resolution and legal consultation may also be needed.

Time-limited trials of treatment are common in pediatric and adolescent medicine and can aid collaborative decision-making by clarifying the benefits and burdens of the treatment. This can then inform decisions about whether to continue or forgo the treatment. However, a child may dissent from the use of a time-limited trial and parents or guardians may refuse them. Even when used, the results of a trial are sometimes unclear. In such cases, the responsible professional should collaborate with the parents or guardians and the patient, as able and willing to be involved, to decide whether to continue the treatment for another time-limited period. The responsible professional should elicit the patient's assent to or dissent from the decision. If the child dissents, the trial generally should not be repeated. Ethics consultation may be needed to address disagreement between the patient and parents or guardians concerning time-limited trials.

## F. Guidelines for Decision-Making with Adolescents

From fourteen years of age onward, the decision-making capacity of adolescents should be respected. As appropriate based on individual assessment, they should be offered opportunities to make informed choices and to participate with their parents or guardians in decisions about their treatment and care.

Adolescence presents a challenge to treatment decision-making. Most adolescents still reasonably expect to be able to rely on adults but may want to make their own decisions about some aspects of their lives. The adolescent patient may feel an urge to defer to the authority of parents or guardians even when he or she believes that parents or guardians are making bad decisions. Adolescents may struggle with the limitations that illness imposes on them, which may include being treated in a children's hospital or on a pediatric floor designed to appeal to the interests and needs of much younger patients. Professionals who specialize in the care of adolescent patients recognize these struggles.

Research from developmental psychology suggests that beginning at about age fourteen, adolescents' problem-solving abilities progressively resemble those of adults, although adults are more likely than adolescents to consider risks and long-term consequences when making medical decisions. An individual assessment of the adolescent patient is essential to determine how capable this patient is of making decisions about medical care, including about life-sustaining treatment, and how interested this patient is in making these decisions.

Failure to provide significant medical information to adolescents (and to older children) is not advisable and can have serious negative consequences. Professionals should be prepared to help parents and guardians who may be reluctant to share health information with an adolescent patient to understand how providing a patient with information relevant to his or her health recognizes the patient as a person. The responsible professional should support the direct involvement of the patient in decision-making and should fulfill the professional's duty of care to the individual patient. On occasion, these responsibilities may require the professional to challenge parents' or guardians' beliefs and wishes out of a duty to the patient.

The responsible professional should support the adolescent patient's decision-making about life-sustaining treatment, including time-limited trials. If there is disagreement among participants concerning life-sustaining interventions, ethics consultation or conflict resolution may be required to address the wishes of the patient. Any decision to oppose the wishes of the adolescent patient or the views of parents or guardians based on the patient's explicit or inferred preferences and values should include ethics consultation and legal consultation.

In recognition of the adolescent's growing autonomy as a person, the adolescent patient's ability to make informed decisions should be supported. At the same time, the still-developing capacities of adolescents should be kept in mind. Parents or guardians of seriously ill adolescents may be highly protective of them, or of their own authority concerning treatment decision-making. If an adolescent was born with a life-threatening or chronic condition or was diagnosed as a young child, parents or guardians have had years of experience making treatment decisions on the child's behalf. They may not see why this should change, even if the adolescent, as the result of years of experience as a patient, may have developed excellent capacity to engage in decision-making. Professionals who care for adolescents should help parents and guardians to recognize how the maturing adolescent differs from the older child with respect to self-determination and how the treatment decision-making process can adapt to the changing psychology, needs, and interests of an older adolescent patient.

As noted above, treatment decisions in the care of adolescent patients may involve time-limited trials. If there is disagreement among participants about whether to undertake a time-limited trial or continue a treatment for another time-limited period, the responsible professional should make sure that the patient's perspective receives great weight. The adolescent patient should be able to request ethics consultation.

## G. Guidelines for Decision-Making by Mature Minors and Emancipated Minors

Health care professionals responsible for the care of adolescent patients should know the laws of the state in which they practice with respect to the decision-making status of mature minors.

Mature minors are older adolescents who are recognized by law as having the ability to make informed decisions about their own health care, although they may still be supervised by parents or guardians. Mature minor statutes typically cover adolescents' ability to give consent to reproductive health services. As statutes and case law concerning emancipated minors and mature minors are state-specific, professionals who treat adolescents should know the laws of the state in which they practice. Ethics consultation may be necessary if state law on medical decision-making by mature minors does not cover the clinical situation at hand or if a mature minor's decision-making capacity is in doubt.

Health care professionals should also know the laws of the state in which they practice with respect to the decision-making of emancipated minors. Emancipated minors should be respected as autonomous persons and decision-makers.

Emancipation is defined by state statute. The term "emancipated minor" tends to refer to adolescents who are not yet legally adults by age, but who live without the supervision of a parent or guardian. These adolescents may have adult responsibilities. They may be married, have children, or live on their own and support themselves. They are still adolescents physiologically and developmentally and may receive medical care in pediatric or adolescent-medicine settings. Adolescents who are emancipated minors by statute have the right to make their own medical decisions if they have decision-making capacity. Ethics consultation may be necessary if an emancipated minor's decision-making capacity is uncertain due to medical or developmental factors.

SECTION 4

# Guidelines for Care Transitions

## Introduction: Care Settings and Care Transitions near the End of Life

In the course of illness, many patients facing decisions about life-sustaining treatment or patients nearing the end of life move between care settings. Patients may be hospitalized to receive some forms of medical treatment or to treat pain, symptoms, treatment side effects, or acute episodes of illness. These patients may also receive care in nonhospital settings, such as a nursing home, the home of the patient or a loved one, or a residential hospice. This section of the *Guidelines* addresses transitions between care settings.

As the result of the hospice movement in the United States, individuals who wish to die at home or in a homelike setting usually have access to a local hospice program that can help them organize their medical and nursing care throughout the dying process. However, practices concerning the timely referral of hospice-eligible patients by health care professionals to hospice programs vary widely across the nation, as does access to residential hospice services for patients who cannot or do not wish to die at home. Health care professionals should be prepared to answer questions from patients and loved ones about hospice referral and hospice programs. For descriptions of the Medicare and Medicaid Hospice Benefits and hospice use across care settings, see Part One, Section 4. For additional guidance on the transition to hospice in the context of cancer care, see Part Three, Section 4G ("Chemotherapy and Other Cancer Treatments").

Nursing home residents should be able to die in the familiar setting of the nursing home if they wish to do so. However, among residents who die in the nursing home setting, hospice enrollment ranges from less than 10 to 30 percent of total deaths.[24] This variation and the relatively low rate of hospice enrollment among nursing home residents near the end of life, relative to hospice enrollment nationally, may reflect a lack of understanding about hospice eligibility among residents and their loved ones. It may also reflect the financial disincentive for nursing homes to encourage hospice enrollment, as Medicare reimbursement rates for hospice beds are lower than rates for Medicare skilled-nursing beds. The Medicare Hospice Benefit may thus be less accessible to this population as compared with other eligible populations, unless nursing homes take the initiative to address equitable access to hospice as a matter of organizational ethics.

There are many ethical challenges involved in transitions between hospital and non-hospital care settings when a patient is facing decisions about life-sustaining treatment or is approaching the end of life. Ethical issues also arise when professionals in different institutions or different locations of a multisite institution must collaborate with one another to provide good care for a patient and prevent harm during care transitions. This section of the *Guidelines* offers guidance for individual professionals and health care teams transferring care of a patient or engaged in discharge planning as this patient faces an illness or condition requiring decisions about life-sustaining treatment or approaches the end of life. Part Two, Section 6E ("Guidelines Supporting Care Transitions") provides guidance concerning the institutional policies and processes that support good care by professionals and teams during care transitions.

This section addresses both hand-offs within institutions and transfers between institutions. Care transitions within an institution involve formal transfers of responsibility (often called "hand-offs") for a patient's care. Hand-offs occur during shift changes and staff rotations, and also occur when a patient moves from the care of one team to another team in the same institution. Hand-offs within an institution are an inevitable feature of patient care and normally do not involve or require explicit decision-making by the patient or surrogate. However, patient transfer from one institution to another, or to home, is a major decision affecting care options and quality of life. It must involve the patient or surrogate. Discharge planning should strive to respect the preferences of patients or decisions of surrogates in keeping with surrogate decision-making standards as described in Part Two, Section 2D ("Surrogate Decision-Making") and discussed further below.

## A. General Guidelines for Hand-Offs between Professionals and Transfers Across Care Settings

### Continuity of care across shift changes

Transfers of responsibility affect all aspects of care when patients face decisions about life-sustaining treatment or approach the end of life. This is true both in hospitals and in nonhospital settings in which medical care, nursing care, or other care must be provided. Nurses are likely to be familiar with transfers of responsibility as this practice is necessitated by shift work, and the profession of nursing has developed protocols for safe hand-offs between nurses during shift changes. In hospitals, the frequency of hand-offs between physicians has increased in recent years. In academic medical centers, mandatory reductions in the number of consecutive hours resident physicians can spend on duty, prompted by concern over fatigue as a cause of human error, have affected the structure of inpatient medical care. Resident physicians now formally sign out at the end of a shift, requiring that responsibility for patient care be handed off to another physician. This structural change has predictably increased discontinuity in patient care. Other physicians, such as those in the newer specialties of adult hospitalists and pediatric hospitalists, also work in shifts and participate in transfers routinely. Hospitalists who care for adults frequently care for Medicare-eligible patients, as these patients are likely to represent a significant portion of a hospital's patient census due to the prevalence of age-associated conditions that may involve medical or surgical treatment available in a hospital setting. This specialty thus plays a pivotal role in continuity of care when a hospitalized patient is facing decisions about life-sustaining treatment or is near the end of life.

Discontinuity in care creates safety hazards and frustrations by increasing opportunities for miscommunication and failure in the transfer of information. Discontinuities also have consequences for physician-patient relationships. A hospitalized patient may have no idea who is in charge of his or her care or may believe that his or her care is being directed by a specific physician who is not, in fact, currently acting in this role.

**Professionals should recognize good hand-offs as sound practice and integral to patient safety and should follow an ethically appropriate process.**

In the care of patients facing decisions about life-sustaining treatment or nearing the end of life, an ethically appropriate hand-off process ensures that each professional who assumes responsibility for a patient's care has access to the following information:

- all diagnostic information and the most recent assessment of the patient's current medical condition;
- treatment directives or other documentation of patient preferences and goals of care established in keeping with these preferences;
- the care plan, including medications, standing medical orders, and the palliative care plan for pain and symptom management and access to supportive services;
- the most recent evaluation of decision-making capacity;
- proxy appointment documents stating the patient's preference for who should assume the role of surrogate if the patient loses decision-making capacity, or other documentation of surrogacy arrangements;
- pending or foreseeable treatment decisions that may occur during this professional's period of responsibility for care;
- psychological, social, spiritual, and family factors that affect this patient's well-being; and
- the identity of the responsible professional—the physician or other health care professional who currently has primary responsibility for the overall care and condition of this patient.

The identity of the responsible professional should also be known to the patient, the surrogate (if any), other loved ones involved in the patient's care, and members of the health care team. Team members should have a reliable means of communicating with this professional.

Transfers of responsibility across care settings require consultation with the patient to respect patient preferences (or with the surrogate applying surrogate decision-making standards) concerning discharge from one setting and admission to another setting, including the home.

The location of care has a profound effect on the type of care a patient receives. Transfers across care settings should be recognized as having a potentially major impact on a patient's care options and quality of life, an impact that may be greater than any individual decision to accept or refuse a particular intervention. This means that transfer decisions must involve the patient or surrogate. Transfers and discharge planning should strive to respect patient preferences or surrogate decisions in keeping with the standards for surrogate decision-making. When this is not possible or the responsible professional is concerned that the care setting preferred by the patient or chosen by the surrogate is not appropriate for the patient in light of his or her care needs, the responsible professional must attempt to resolve these differences through discussion. Ethics consultation, conflict resolution, or both may be necessary.

When transfers of responsibility occur across care settings, professionals should recognize that their duty of care extends to the safe arrival of the patient and information at the destination.

Poor transfers can undo good decisions and good care. To minimize discontinuities in care, professionals responsible for the transfer of patients between care settings or for the discharge of hospitalized patients should recognize that their own duty of care extends to their patient's safe arrival at the destination and to completing a good transfer to the next caregiver.

This duty may require professionals to resolve known problems in a patient's care prior to a transfer or discharge, including conflicts over treatment decisions. Even if the problem cannot be resolved definitively prior to a transfer or discharge, it is better to try to resolve it rather than to permit an acknowledged problem to travel with a patient and continue to affect the patient's care. It is unacceptable to use transfers and discharges to turf known problems in a patient's care to other professionals and other care settings or to foist unresolved problems on paraprofessionals or family caregivers who may lack the authority or ability to resolve care problems.

The duty of care also requires professionals to follow sound processes for the transfer of records and information. (See Part Two, Section 6.)

## B. Guidelines on Care Transitions for Nursing Home Residents

### The nursing home as an end-of-life care setting

In the United States, two-thirds of deaths resulting from end-stage dementia and associated comorbidities occur in nursing homes.[25] The nursing home is an end-of-life care setting for these residents, and also for residents with end-stage cancer or with advanced chronic disease affecting major organ systems. As many nursing home residents are elderly and frail, they may be highly susceptible to infection, bone fractures, and other serious health problems. The nursing home may therefore become an end-of-life care setting for residents whose overall health is deteriorating. According to the National Nursing Home Survey, the average length of stay in a nursing home is less than two years for residents on Medicaid and less than one year for all residents before transfer to the hospital.[26]

The reality that most nursing home residents, due to their age and their medical condition, are near the end of their lives (and may, in some cases, be dying) exists in tension with the way nursing homes are regulated and organized.[27] The landmark Omnibus Budget Reconciliation Act (OBRA) of 1987 rejected the use of nursing homes as warehouses for the elderly and led to efforts to improve the quality of care and the lives of residents. OBRA '87 reoriented nursing homes toward rehabilitative and restorative care that would maintain or improve residents' functional status. However, the goals of rehabilitative and restorative care may conflict with the goals of good care near the end of life. When a dying person's functional status is deteriorating due to an underlying disease process, efforts to maintain or restore function can no longer help this person and may cause harm.

Nursing home leaders and other staff members may be aware of a tension between regulatory goals and the real needs of residents who are dying, but they may not be sure what to do about it. Regulations can have unintended consequences by focusing on task-oriented care rather than patient-centered care. The desire to avoid "deficiency" ratings during each nursing home's annual survey by regulators may therefore orient care toward survey performance and away from the preferences and best interests of residents who are dying.

For example, weight loss is one of the sentinel events that nursing homes must report, and that, if reported, will be investigated by surveyors. Weight loss in a nursing home resident could be a sign of substandard care but could also be a sign that a well-cared-for resident is near the end of life, when a loss of interest in eating and drinking is common. If staff members fail to recognize that a resident is losing weight because the dying process is under way, they may attempt to fix the perceived problem (weight loss) by interventions that cannot reverse this process and may result in discomfort or other burdens to the dying person. Such interventions may also be contrary to the resident's preferences, as well as evidence-based best practices. Extensive research shows that the practice of placing feeding tubes in nursing home residents with advanced dementia fails to confer benefit while inflicting significant burdens. For dying residents, this effort may cause harm. For additional material, see Part Three, Section 1C, "Discussing Values Concerning Nutrition and Hydration," and Part Three, Section 4F, "Nutrition and Hydration," and the Bibliography supporting these subsections.

### Transfer to the hospital should not be used to avoid end-of-life decision-making and care in nursing homes.

Avoiding advance care planning, and then turfing dying people and decisions about their care, is contrary to the ethical goals reflected in these *Guidelines* and to widely recognized patient safety and quality improvement goals. Transfers may be uncomfortable, confusing, or stressful to the dying person and may be also be confusing to the person's loved ones. Transfers, which may occur repeatedly for some nursing home residents, introduce serious discontinuities into care, each with the potential for miscommunication, medication errors, and other mistakes. Empirical research into regional variation in transfers from nursing homes to hospitals concludes that in regions with high rates of cost-shifting transfers ("churning"), a nursing home resident with advanced dementia faces a high risk of having a feeding tube placed, despite ample evidence that this practice is likely to burden and even harm this patient without offering benefit.[28]

Retaining a dying resident and addressing decisions about life-sustaining treatment may seem inherently risky to nursing home professionals. While some transfers to the hospital can be justified based on the medical needs of a nursing home resident, transferring dying nursing home residents because they are dying can become a strategy for avoiding a perceived risk to the facility. It may also reflect a missed opportunity for conducting advance care planning upon admission, including consideration of a resident's preferences and advance directives. Efforts to develop cost-effective models of palliative care and end-of-life care for nursing homes and for specific nursing home populations, such as residents with advanced dementia, have the potential to improve continuity of care by reducing the need for hospital transfers. These models may also help establish a philosophy of care within the nursing home that can coexist with the rehabilitative model but is more appropriate for the needs of those residents who are near the end of life. The Bibliography for this section includes relevant material. The websites included in the Bibliography offer further resources.

Nursing home medical directors and directors of nursing should clarify the medical conditions or other circumstances that would justify a decision to transfer a dying nursing home resident to the hospital.

In view of the burdens and potential harms associated with transfers, nursing home leaders have an ethical obligation to identify the situations in which the benefits of transfer would exceed the burdens and therefore justify transfer. They should also address how dying patients will be cared for in the nursing home when they will not be transferred because transfer is likely to contribute no benefit or is likely to result in harm. Nursing home staff members may have differing perceptions of the burdens and benefits of transferring dying patients or may have concerns or liability-related fears about the medically appropriate course of action when a nursing home resident is dying. Staff education and opportunities for ethical reflection are essential.

Nursing home medical directors and directors of nursing should be familiar with outcomes data on attempting CPR in the nursing home setting and should clarify evidence-based practice for all staff.

Studies of outcomes data following attempted cardiopulmonary resuscitation have found that the poorest outcomes are associated with CPR attempts involving elderly nursing home residents and elderly persons living in the community, due to their underlying health conditions and other factors.[29] In one study, which found that nearly all nursing home residents who were transferred to the hospital following a CPR attempt were pronounced dead on arrival or died within a few days of admission, rates of survival to discharge ranged from 11 percent among community residents to below 2 percent among nursing home residents, with extremely poor health status among nursing home residents who survived to discharge.[30] These data strongly suggest that CPR should be recognized as a marginally beneficial intervention in certain settings and within certain populations. To prevent harms to residents, health care professionals who work in these settings have a duty to clarify evidence-based practice for staff.

Integrating portable medical orders based on the Physician Orders for Life-Sustaining Treatment (POLST) Paradigm (described in Part Two, Section 4C, below) into advance care planning in nursing homes and training staff in their appropriate use—so they are aware of residents' wishes concerning CPR and other interventions—are additional steps nursing home leaders can take in jurisdictions where a POLST-type program is available. Nursing home leaders in any jurisdiction can also proactively collaborate with local emergency departments and other first responders on education for staff and trained volunteers (such as firefighters and ambulance corps members in some communities) to clarify situations in which emergency responders should not be called because a nursing home resident has elected to forgo CPR. Education can also clarify good practice for situations in which emergency responders are called to a nursing home.

For additional guidance, see Part Two, Section 4C ("Guidelines on Portable Medical Orders") and Part Three, Section 4D ("Cardiopulmonary Resuscitation and Cardiac Treatments").

**Nursing home staff should discuss the goals of nursing home care with residents and surrogates on admission and should document treatment preferences and write the necessary medical orders. Staff education should address the proper use of advance directives and portable medical orders. Residents and surrogates should receive accurate information about the effectiveness of interventions in nursing home populations.**

Residents enter nursing homes from different places, and their prior experience with advance care planning will vary. Given the likelihood that nursing home residents or their surrogates will need to make decisions about life-sustaining treatment, initiating advance care planning and then using those documents in ongoing care planning should be priorities for nursing home medical directors and nursing directors. Staff knowledge of advance directives may be weak. Education and guidance in the use of advance directives and in processes to document residents' treatment preferences such as portable medical orders (described in Part Two, Section 4C, below) are integral to preventing miscommunication and the initiation of treatment that may be unwanted or ineffective.

As part of advance care planning conducted in the nursing home setting, residents and surrogates should receive accurate information about interventions that may be significantly less effective in this setting and about any alternatives that may better reflect a resident's preferences and support this resident's goals of care.

Professionals responsible for the care of nursing home residents should recognize their role in end-of-life care and recognize the nursing home as an end-of-life care setting.

Nursing home leaders should provide nursing home medical directors, physicians, nurses, and other staff with opportunities to develop the competencies described in Part One, Section 2. Collaboration with clinician education programs at local hospitals and with local hospice programs may aid ethics education concerning the care of patients who may transfer between care settings and may help identify local end-of-life resources, such as hospice, that should be available to these patients.

## C. Guidelines on Portable Medical Orders

Portable medical orders support good care near the end of life by providing explicit guidance for likely medical scenarios in the form of documents that can accompany this patient across care settings, including home, hospital, nursing home, and hospice. A set of portable medical orders is often referred to as a "POLST" if it is the product of a care planning program based on the Physician Orders for Life-Sustaining Treatment (POLST) Paradigm, described below. An order concerning a specific intervention, such as a DNR order, also constitutes a portable order when it travels with the patient to be honored across care settings.

The following three guidelines concern the preparation and use of portable medical orders by individual professionals, both within and across care settings:

Professionals in any setting who are responsible for the care of patients who may be near the end of life should know how to communicate and collaborate with patients to write portable medical orders to address potential treatments in response to medical emergencies, including but not limited to cardiopulmonary resuscitation.

Professionals who are responsible for the care of patients who may be near the end of life should know how to use portable medical orders within and across care settings. Institutions that provide care near the end of life and organizations that provide emergency medical services should provide training and policy guidance for their personnel concerning the use of portable medical orders.

Institutional processes for advance care planning and for discharge planning should provide for the regular review of all existing documentation, including medical orders, and should aim to include the preparation of portable medical orders that can accompany patients across care settings and to their destination.

In the United States, the POLST Paradigm is a standardized process for discussing patient preferences and establishing a care plan that travels with the patient.[31] Health care providers and policy-makers can adapt the POLST Paradigm for use at the state or community level. By identifying and documenting a patient's current goals and treatment preferences and by translating these goals into medical orders whenever possible, this process aims to promote continuity of care and to reduce the potential for harm resulting from confusion, delay, or unwanted interventions. A benefit of the POLST Paradigm is that it is designed to be honored by emergency medical personnel and others who need explicit guidance when responding to a medical emergency. The Bibliography includes information about the POLST Paradigm, including studies of its use in different states and jurisdictions. The POLST Paradigm consists of three essential steps for health care professionals to follow:

1.  Initiate a discussion of the treatment preferences of a seriously ill patient—with the patient or with the surrogate if the patient lacks decision-making capacity—with reference to the patient's current condition and to the medical emergencies that may result from this condition.
2.  Document emergency medical orders in keeping with patient preferences or surrogate decision-making using a distinctive, standardized form.
3.  Honor these orders across care settings and review these orders whenever the patient or surrogate wishes to discuss them, the patient's condition changes, or the patient is transferred to a different care setting.

The goals of the POLST Paradigm are similar to the goals of an advance care planning process. A key difference is that the POLST Paradigm is designed for patients who may face transfer in an emergency, while advance care planning may be initiated well before this point and may address a broader range of circumstances. Another key difference is that only patients may write advance directives, but either patients or the surrogates of patients who lack decision-making capacity can use the POLST Paradigm.

The preparation of portable medical orders should include discussion and review of care planning already completed by the patient or surrogate, so that any new or revised orders can be added to the patient's current care plan. Portable medical orders should also specify whether the patient has a surrogate and should provide contact information for the surrogate.

Portable medical orders typically include explicit guidance reflecting patient preferences or surrogate decisions with respect to emergency interventions such as cardiopulmonary resuscitation or intubation and the preferred level of care and interventions at the patient's destination. Alternatively, the portable document created through a POLST-type process can simply direct medical personnel to contact the patient or (if the patient does not have decision-making capacity) the surrogate named in the document.

Documentation of medical orders to cover future emergencies does not supplant the decision-making authority of a patient or surrogate. The document is intended to be recognized as a reliable and recent record of the patient's preferences for care or the surrogate's decisions if the patient has lost decision-making capacity. However, a patient may change his or her mind, especially as the patient's condition changes, or a surrogate may conclude that treatment decisions need to be altered as the patient's condition changes.

If a patient with decision-making capacity subsequently loses decision-making capacity, the physician or other professional responsible for the patient's care should be prepared to work with the patient's surrogate to review the patient's explicit preferences, or (if those are not known) the patient's values and preferences as best the surrogate can infer them, or (if those too are unknown) the patient's best interests. The professional and surrogate should apply the standards for surrogate decision-making detailed in Part Two, Section 2D ("Surrogate Decision-Making"):

- If the patient's physical condition has deteriorated and the professional and the patient's surrogate agree that the goals of care should be changed, with the surrogate applying the standards for surrogate decision-making, the professional responsible for the patient's care writes new orders to reflect the revised care plan and cover any medical contingencies not already addressed.
- If the patient's physical condition has not deteriorated, but there is evidence that the patient's preferences concerning life-sustaining interventions are changing or are inconsistent (for example, if a patient has begun to refuse dialysis on some days but not on others), the preferences documented in a set of portable medical orders prepared while the patient still had decision-making capacity should be carefully reviewed with the surrogate. Ethics consultation may be necessary to resolve conflicts between the patient's previously documented preferences and current apparent preferences.
- If the patient's surrogate, applying the standards for surrogate decision-making, believes that the patient should receive emergency interventions different from those reflected in portable medical orders completed while the patient had decision-making capacity, the responsible professional should ask why the surrogate believes the patient would have wanted the documented orders to be changed. The surrogate may be concerned that the patient did not consider the current clinical scenario or would now decide differently than the decision reflected in the portable medical orders. Deviating from medical orders created when the patient had decision-making capacity requires careful consideration and may require ethics consultation.

Because the POLST Paradigm is a model that is adapted by individual states or communities, professionals who work with portable medical orders should be familiar with relevant state law and policy. Professionals should know how to obtain guidance within their institution concerning the proper use of a POLST document or other types of portable medical order authorized for use in their jurisdiction and care setting.

For related guidance, see Part Two, Section 1; Part Two, Sections 2D and 2F ("Surrogate Decision-Making" and "Documenting the Decision"); and Part Two, Section 6D ("Guidelines Supporting the Use of Portable Medical Orders") .

## D. Guidelines on Discharge Planning and Collaboration with Nursing Homes, Home Care, Hospice, and Outpatient Care

A hospitalized patient who is terminally ill, but whose medical condition and goals of care no longer require the patient to remain hospitalized, needs a discharge plan that can be maintained at the patient's destination by a caregiving team that may include professionals, paraprofessionals, family members, and other loved ones, as well as the patient, as able. An ethically sound discharge plan is one that addresses established and foreseeable needs and has a reasonable prospect of working in practice, including under less than optimal conditions. While a patient's medical condition may require that readmission to the hospital be considered in the future, the possibility of readmission should not be used as a substitute for a sound discharge plan. Such a plan is always needed.

**Professionals involved in discharge planning should recognize an ethical obligation to create sound plans.**

Creating discharge plans is a professional responsibility. The actions of the professional responsible for the patient's care at the time of discharge and of other professionals on the health care team affect the integrity of the discharge plan. These team members should be prepared to collaborate with staff members (such as social workers or nurse-managers) who may have formal responsibility for discharge planning in an institution. Discharge planning should also involve community professionals who are already involved in the patient's care, such as primary care providers, home care providers, and hospice providers. In some cases, a hospice provider will have primary responsibility for the discharge plan if the patient will receive hospice services at his or her destination.

A discharge plan omitting information relevant to the patient's needs, anticipated problems, goals of care, and follow-up care is not an ethically sound plan. Professionals using paper or electronic discharge planning systems should recognize their responsibility for the transfer of information to the patient's destination as part of their own duty of care. System-level improvements to ensure that a discharge summary cannot be processed without required information may reduce such errors of omission.

**Discharge planning should include the review of all existing documentation and should aim to include the preparation of portable medical orders to address any foreseeable medical emergencies.**

Portable medical orders are appropriate for care transitions involving seriously ill patients and can help ensure that a patient or surrogate's treatment decisions will be known and honored in emergency situations. They should be reviewed with the patient or surrogate both at the discharging institution (where any errors can be corrected before discharge) and at the receiving institution or other destination, where they can be converted into standing orders.

Discharge planning should aim to follow the preferences and meet the needs of patients in light of the capacities of prospective future caregivers. It is important to identify the reasonable accommodations and means of assistance that can sustain the discharge plan.

Patients may have strong preferences about where they receive care for many reasons, including the reality that the location of care affects treatment options. As discussed, discharge planning must take patient preferences concerning the location of care and other elements of the discharge plan into account. Sometimes a patient may express a preference for a discharge plan that the responsible professional believes will not be sustainable in view of the patient's medical condition or other factors. For example, a frail elderly patient may express a preference to go home from the hospital and may refuse to consider a nursing home placement recommended by the responsible professional because the patient is confident that loved ones will be able to function as caregivers. However, the patient's loved ones may not feel they can safely and adequately meet the patient's care needs. The responsible professional should try to ensure the feasibility of the discharge plan. Whenever the patient's preferred discharge plan cannot be put into effect, the responsible professional must explain this to the patient and discuss alternatives. Ethics consultation may be needed.

An interdisciplinary approach to discharge planning can help the patient and caregivers reach consensus on a sustainable discharge plan or on a time-limited trial of a plan that reflects the patient's preferences but whose sustainability is uncertain, with identification of a sustainable backup plan. Involving a social worker or another team member with expert knowledge of institutional and community resources to collaborate in developing a discharge plan may help patients, family members, and other loved ones identify and discuss options.

Discharge planning for patients who need ongoing pain and symptom management should include a team member with palliative care expertise to ensure continuity of care at the patient's destination.

Discharge planning must integrate palliative care into care near the end of life, including pain and symptom management plus access to supportive services such as mental health care, chaplaincy, and social work. Whether or not they wish to enroll in hospice, patients forgoing life-sustaining treatment or nearing the end of life should have a discharge plan that reflects their current palliative care needs, gives them ongoing access to expert palliative care services, and minimizes the likelihood of hospital readmission due to uncontrolled pain and symptoms or inadequate social supports. Discharge planning for these patients should include a consultation with a member of the palliative care team, such as a nurse who has expert knowledge of palliative care delivery outside of the inpatient setting.

The palliative care consultation can also identify complex palliative care needs, such as those involving pediatric patients or patients with psychiatric histories, which may require additional specialist consultations prior to discharge.

## Continuity of palliative care during discharge to nursing home

Approximately 45 percent of nursing home residents are admitted from an acute-care hospital or a hospital-based skilled nursing facility.[32] Nursing home medical and nursing staff should therefore expect to collaborate with hospital professionals regularly. While patients discharged to nursing homes may have palliative care needs, nursing homes may not have well-established palliative care programs. To ensure the adequacy of each patient's discharge plan, a member of the patient's hospital team who has palliative care expertise should contact the professional who will be responsible for the patient's care following discharge to review the patient's ongoing needs for pain and symptom management and to determine how these needs can be met in the nursing home. The hospital-based palliative care specialist should be familiar with payment mechanisms for palliative care in nursing homes, as these details may not be known to patients and loved ones or to staff in nursing homes that do not yet have an established palliative care program.

In addition to collaborating with hospital discharge planners, nursing home medical directors and nursing directors should be familiar with models for delivering palliative care in nursing homes and should advocate for the use of these models in their own institutions.

## Continuity of palliative care during discharge to home care

Patients who need ongoing pain and symptom management, and also some level of home health services, should have a discharge plan that provides palliative care. Some hospitals offer home care through their palliative care program or through a clinical case management program, while some home health agencies and hospice programs offer palliative care in addition to other services. The palliative care specialist and the social worker on the patient's health care team should identify and collaborate with the home care or hospice providers in the community where the patient will live following discharge to ensure that the discharge plan incorporates all services needed by the patient.

Home care programs that provide pain and symptom management or other clinical services may not offer the range of supportive care services that may be available to patients and families through hospice. However, some patients who need both palliative care and home care may not yet be hospice-eligible. Others may be hospice-eligible but prefer to continue treatment aimed at cure or long-term survival, or prefer not to enroll in hospice for some other reason. The palliative care consultation for these patients should include an assessment of the patient's needs and current resources for palliative care, including mental health care and spiritual care, as well as the supportive care needs of loved ones. The discharge plan should identify ways to address these needs once the patient is discharged and the home care plan is in place.

The palliative care consultation for a patient who is being discharged to home care, and for any terminally ill patient with ongoing palliative care needs, should include the option of hospice. The patient and loved ones should be confident that the option to enroll in hospice remains open.

### Continuity of palliative care during discharge to hospice

A patient's options for hospice care may vary by region, medical management needs, family circumstances, and patient preferences. The palliative care specialist and the social worker on the patient's health care team should familiarize themselves with the hospice programs serving the community where the patient will live following discharge. Professionals responsible for discharge planning should be prepared to discuss different options with the patient or surrogate if more than one option for hospice exists. Discharge to hospice will also allow consideration of how hospice can support the patient's family and other loved ones in their care of the patient and in coping with the patient's condition.

## E. Guidelines on Care Transitions for Patients Who Will Die in the Hospital

Some hospitalized patients who are expected to die shortly—often following a decision to forgo further life-sustaining treatment—cannot safely be discharged or transferred due to the stress and potential harms of transport. Other dying patients have pain and symptoms that would be difficult or impossible to manage outside of an ICU or other inpatient setting. Some do not have a home where needed care can be organized quickly and provided continuously until death. All of these patients need to receive good end-of-life care in the hospital from professionals with appropriate expertise. Transfer should not be forced on these patients or their loved ones.

Professionals in the emergency department or another unit in the hospital who are responsible for the care of a patient who is expected to die shortly should be prepared to care for this patient in the hospital.

End-of-life care in the hospital may sometimes need to be provided in a critical care setting due to a patient's condition. For example, some patients whose condition is deteriorating will present in the emergency department with poorly controlled symptoms. Whenever possible, the dying patient should be moved to a room that offers privacy and quiet for the patient and loved ones. If responsibility for patient care will change hands during this care transition, the responsible professional should follow an ethically sound transfer process as described above.

The care plan for a patient who is dying in the hospital should provide for ongoing relief of pain and symptoms and access to other supportive services that may be needed by the patient or loved ones.

The palliative care plan for a patient dying in the hospital may include moving the patient to an inpatient hospice unit, if available and feasible. In hospitals where inpatient hospice care is not available to a patient who is expected to die soon, the professional currently responsible for the patient's care should ensure that the patient's care plan includes all medical orders needed by the medical and nursing staff to manage pain and symptoms around the clock. The care plan should reflect patient preferences concerning end-of-life care. If the patient's health care team does not already include a specialist in palliative care, the responsible professional should consult with the hospital's palliative care service to update the care plan and ensure ongoing relief of pain and symptoms. The responsible professional should also take steps to ensure that the patient and loved ones have access to chaplaincy or other supportive services that may be desired.

For additional guidance relevant to the care of the dying patient in the hospital, including situations in which palliative care must be initiated in the emergency department, see Part Three, Sections 4A and 4J, "(Forgoing Life-Sustaining Treatments: Ethical and Practical Considerations for Clinicians" and "Palliative Sedation")."

SECTION 5

# Guidelines for the Determination of Death

## Introduction

According to the Uniform Determination of Death Act (UDDA):

> "An individual who has sustained either (1) irreversible cessation of circulatory
> and respiratory functions, or (2) irreversible cessation of all functions of the entire
> brain, including the brain stem, is dead. A determination of death must be made in
> accordance with accepted medical standards." (See Cited Legal Authorities.)

The UDDA was adopted in 1980 by the National Conference of Commissioners on
Uniform State Laws. It is not itself a statute, but was formulated as a model statute for
states to consider. In 1981, the President's Commission for the Study of Ethical Problems
in Medicine and Biomedical and Behavioral Research issued a report, *Defining Death*, that
recognized medical standards for determining and declaring death and that encouraged all
states to adopt the UDDA.[33] A majority of states now use the UDDA language in their
statutes. The small number of states that do not have a brain-death statute may embrace
brain death as a means of determining death by case law or regulation. These *Guidelines*
also use the UDDA standard for the determination of death.

The UDDA expanded the criteria for recognizing that death—the loss of integrated
functioning of the organism—had occurred. Under the expanded criteria, a determination
of death could be made according to *either* circulatory and respiratory criteria *or* neurological criteria. The development of technologies such as electroencephalograms (EEGs) and
brain perfusion studies enabled clinicians to determine that death by neurological criteria (commonly called "brain death") had occurred even when mechanical ventilation and
other technologies maintained the body's cardiopulmonary systems.

Discussing death by neurological criteria with the loved ones of a deceased patient may be challenging, due to what they are seeing: a body that still looks like that of a living person. As long as the body's organs are being perfused, the body will remain warm, the skin will keep its normal color, and the heart will continue to beat. As long as mechanical ventilation continues, the body will appear to be breathing. Clinicians caring for grieving families must be careful both to clarify that death by neurological criteria *is* death—that the patient has already died—and to distinguish death by neurological criteria from neurological states in which a patient is unresponsive but alive. For additional guidance on discussing brain injuries and neurological states, see Part Three, Section 4.

## A. Procedural Guidelines for Making a Determination of Death and for Making a Declaration of Death

### Use of medical standards in determining and declaring death

The responsible professional should make the determination of death in accordance with standards of medical practice at the time of the assessment.

All states recognize circulatory and respiratory criteria for determining death: When the responsible professional determines that the patient has experienced an irreversible cessation of circulatory and respiratory functions, the patient is declared dead. All states also recognize neurological criteria for determining death, either by statute, case law, or regulation: When the responsible professional determines that the patient has experienced an irreversible cessation of all functions of the entire brain, the patient is declared dead. All professionals should know the law of the state in which they practice.

### Obligation to conduct a neurological evaluation to determine death by neurological criteria

As soon as the responsible professional has a reasonable suspicion that irreversible cessation of all functions of the entire brain, including the brain stem, has occurred, the professional should perform the appropriate bedside tests and procedures to determine the patient's neurological status.[34] Conducting this evaluation does not depend on whether a patient's loved ones want to continue treatment or on the patient's status as a potential organ donor.

### Obligation to make a declaration of death

When a patient meets *either* circulatory and respiratory *or* neurological criteria for a determination of death, the patient should be declared dead by the professional who has made the determination of death. The declaration of death does not require the consent of a surrogate or another person.

### Health care professionals who should not make the declaration of death

The health care professional who makes the declaration of death should:

- not be a member of the organ transplant team, if any, planning or seeking to remove the patient's organs;

- not be a member of the patient's family;
- not be defending a malpractice claim or other formal complaint related to this patient; and
- not have any other special interest in the declaration of the patient's death, such as standing to inherit under the patient's will.

## Communication with loved ones about the determination of death

The professional responsible for making the determination of death and declaring a patient dead is also responsible for explaining to the patient's loved ones that the patient has died and how that has been determined. If death has been determined by neurological criteria, the responsible professional should state that the patient has already died and that the technologies that are maintaining cardiopulmonary and other organ function are not sustaining life. Terms such as "life support," or the suggestion that the patient is being "kept alive by machines," should be avoided in this context, as unclear or inaccurate language may lead loved ones to conclude that the patient is still alive. Subsequent efforts to explain that the patient has died and to withdraw mechanical support may lead to mistrust and anger if loved ones believe that the health care team is "giving up" on a living patient.

To help prevent confusion that may contribute to distress and conflict, professionals working in end-of-life care settings should continually reinforce the importance of clear, accurate, and consistent language with team members and other unit staff, including those who are not directly responsible for a patient's care but may have informal conversations with loved ones after a patient has died.

## Accommodating religious objections to the determination of death by neurological criteria

Some religious groups, including some Orthodox Jews, do not acknowledge death by neurological criteria and recognize only death by circulatory and respiratory criteria. Due to the diversity of American society, health care professionals may encounter a range of religious beliefs and practices concerning death, including religious objections to a determination of death by neurological criteria.

Sometimes loved ones will react to the determination of death by neurological criteria using religious-sounding language (for example, "we're still praying for a miracle") that *may or may not* constitute an objection based in the tenets of a particular religious tradition. This language may indicate a belief that the patient is still alive or reflect an inability to acknowledge that death has already occurred.

Acknowledging religious objections to the declaration of death, including objections to neurological criteria for a determination of death, does not alter the physiological state of the deceased patient. A religious objection to a determination of death by neurological criteria can be accommodated by allowing a delay in the declaration of death or a delay in the cessation of ventilation and any other technologies. The involvement of a board-certified chaplain with experience caring for bereaved families from a variety of religious backgrounds (including but not limited to Christian, Jewish, Islamic, Buddhist, and Hindu faith traditions) and who is familiar with how grief and other emotions may be expressed in religious terms may be helpful in such situations. The chaplain should become involved as soon as the responsible professional has a reasonable suspicion that brain death has occurred.

### Reasonable accommodations involving the delayed withdrawal of treatment following the determination of death by neurological criteria

If a patient's loved ones are not yet able to acknowledge that brain death has occurred, they may resist initial efforts to withdraw what they continue to view as "life support." Some loved ones may acknowledge that brain death has occurred but would like to have time for another loved one to arrive before the machines are disconnected. Delaying the withdrawal of some or all supports for a clearly specified period of time is a reasonable accommodation to help bereaved loved ones begin to adjust to their loss. These reasonable requests should be accommodated if possible.

During this period, the responsible professional and other members of the health care team should continue to clarify that the patient has died and that it is the patient's loved ones who are being cared for. If the determination of death was made in the emergency department or a critical care unit, the patient's body should be moved to a more private space, both to provide privacy for loved ones and to signal that life-saving interventions are no longer possible. The involvement of a chaplain, mental health professional, or other team member with appropriate skills may be helpful in caring for bereaved loved ones during the accommodation period and during the cessation of all mechanical supports at the end of this period. An ethics consultation or other conflict resolution intervention may be necessary if loved ones request that the accommodations be continued beyond the specified period or propose accommodations, such as the introduction of new treatment or a request for a transfer to a different institution, despite the fact that the patient is already dead.

### Cessation of mechanical support after a declaration of death

Once the responsible professional has progressed from making a determination to making a formal declaration of death, all medical interventions should ordinarily cease. Mechanical ventilation and other interventions may temporarily remain in place after a patient has been declared dead when efforts are being made to use the patient's body or body parts for the purposes stated in the state law equivalent of the Uniform Anatomical Gift Act, such as transplantation. (See Cited Legal Authorities.) For additional guidance on discussing organ donation in the context of treatment withdrawal, see Part Three, Section 4A ("Forgoing Life-Sustaining Treatments: Ethical and Practical Considerations for Clinicians").

## B. The Determination of Death: Continuing Ethical Debates

### Organ donation after cardiac (or circulatory) death

The recognition of neurological criteria for the determination of death, through adoption of laws modeled on the UDDA, has permitted a declaration of death followed by the continued perfusion of transplantable organs for a limited time. This allows the organs to remain viable if the donor, while alive, elected organ donation or if the deceased person's loved ones are considering organ donation. Clinical, ethical, and legal standards for the transplantation of vital organs have evolved to protect three entities: the donor, the recipient, and the organs themselves, which constitute an extremely limited resource. One area of remaining controversy, however, concerns cases involving organ donation after cardiac death (DCD) rather than after death declared by neurological criteria. (Some commentators now use the term "donation after circulatory death.")

As stated in the Uniform Anatomical Gift Act (UAGA), a model statute widely adopted by states, the "dead donor rule" requires that a donor be declared dead before vital organs are removed. Some ethical debates have arisen concerning cases in which a catastrophically injured organ donor, who is not dead by neurological criteria and is projected to die shortly after life-sustaining interventions are withdrawn, has been declared dead using circulatory and respiratory criteria after the withdrawal of cardiopulmonary support, and their organs then harvested. Some have questioned whether the cessation of cardiopulmonary function in this scenario (that is, withdrawing cardiopulmonary support followed by cardiac arrest) is truly "irreversible," as required under the UDDA for a declaration of death so that organs can be removed for transplant. Ethical questions have also arisen concerning what constitutes an adequate informed consent process for a surrogate facing the decision to stop life-sustaining treatment and thus allow organ harvest under these circumstances. A decision to stop life-sustaining treatment must be made on its own grounds, following the standards for surrogate decision-making as discussed in Part Two, Section 2D ("Surrogate Decision-Making"), and should be made separately from a decision about organ donation. Careful attention to the informed consent process for DCD is essential, so that the possibility of organ donation does not influence a surrogate's decision about life-sustaining treatment. The surrogate and other loved ones should also be confident that the patient's death is not being hastened out of a desire to harvest the patient's organs.

As the typical patient in this situation is in a critical care setting, the separation of the patient care team from the organ procurement team and the organ transplant team is of ethical importance to ensure that the patient care team is able to remain attentive to the needs of the patient and loved ones and to avoid role confusion between teams with different goals. Education and support for bedside staff involved in the care of a patient during decision-making about DCD is also of ethical and practical importance, as staff may be uncertain how DCD differs from organ donation following a determination of death by neurological criteria, or even how organ donation is permissible under these circumstances.

Ethics education in clinical settings can provide opportunities for professionals to discuss these and other questions and to reflect on their own concerns. The Bibliography for this section includes a selection from the literature on these issues. Part Three, Section 4A and 4B and the Bibliography supporting that section include relevant material and citations on organ donation and on neurological states.

# Guidelines for Institutional Policy

## The Ethical Importance of Good Policy

The values, priorities, and structure of a health care institution affect the lives of the patients, loved ones, and professionals in this institution. Much as professionals have ethical obligations, institutions have ethical responsibilities, too. A growing literature on organizational ethics in health care addresses those institutional responsibilities. Policies and administrative processes can help ensure that an institution's activities are morally acceptable and that its interests and practices are aligned with the interests of its patients. When an institution's patient care policy is carefully and transparently developed, clearly explained, regularly reviewed, and equitably implemented, professionals can confidently rely on that policy. An institution's business decisions—how it protects its operating margin, invests and distributes its resources, and handles its contractual obligations—should be consistent with its obligations to its patients, reflecting a common understanding that health care is a social good that is also a business, and is never merely a business.

When an institution's policy fails to address the moral dimensions of patient care, staff may become confused or demoralized, and patients may be harmed or suffer in other ways. Institutions that are unclear about good (and bad) outcomes of normal work, including health care work, are environments that are not as safe they could be. Educational gaps—for example, between what health care professionals think they know about law on treatment decision-making and end-of-life care and actual law and policy—also have consequences for patient safety and well-being.

The ethical content of a health care institution's policy derives from a range of sources. These include the values of health care ethics and organizational ethics; policy recommendations from relevant professional organizations or groups; trends or consensus on practice within health care professions; the health care needs of the populations an institution serves; and laws, regulations, and standards. An institution's policy is also shaped by the core values it formally affirms—including the words on the wall of the institution's main lobby or the home page of its website—and whether these values are evident in everyday practice.

Policy is shaped by an institution's larger organizational identity as well. An academic medical center, a community hospital, a for-profit long-term care facility, a hospice program, and a home care agency provide care for patients who face decisions about life-sustaining treatment or are nearing the end of life. Some of these institutions may serve the same patients. The obligations, professional affiliations, and business operations of these institutions differ. However, quality and continuity of care is a shared ethical concern with consequences for operations. Because these different types of institutions will need to collaborate to ensure that community members receive good care near the end of life, they need strong policies on continuity of care that can work in practice as patients move among institutions.

Good care near the end of life involves professionals who function both as individuals and as members of teams. Ethically competent professionals rely on ethically sound systems to support the care they provide. This section of these *Guidelines* addresses those aspects of policy within and across institutions that support the professional practices that are the focus of the previous sections of Part Two, on advance care planning (Section 1), treatment decision-making (Section 2), pediatric decision-making and care (Section 3), care transitions (Section 4), and the determination of death (Section 5).

## A. Guidelines on Ethics Services in Institutions Providing Care for Patients Facing Decisions about Life-Sustaining Treatment or Approaching the End of Life

As a practical activity, *clinical ethics* refers to the individuals and processes involved in identifying, analyzing, discussing, and resolving moral dilemmas in the delivery of health care.[35] It is a form of applied ethics, and applies substantive principles, such as the ethical goals outlined in Part One.

The quality of an institution's ethics service will be determined by its competence with respect to the issues that are addressed throughout these *Guidelines*. Improving care for patients confronting decisions about life-sustaining treatment or nearing the end of life requires an institutional commitment to improving the quality of its ethics services. (Since 1992, The Joint Commission, formerly known as the Joint Commission on Accreditation of Healthcare Organizations [JCAHO], has mandated that accredited health care organizations provide some mechanism for addressing ethical concerns.) A robust ethics program shows that an institution takes moral concerns in health care seriously. It shows that an institution makes time and provides structure for ethical reflection and practical guidance on individual cases, for developing ethically sound policy, and for strengthening clinical practice. By contrast, a weak ethics program can do harm. When "ethics" is viewed as just another committee, or as simply a crisis-response team, the effort to integrate ethical competence into clinical practice suffers, and the consequences can be poor care for patients.

Clinical ethics is practiced at the bedside, both when individual professionals strive to do the right thing in their practice and when a professional, patient, loved one, or other person involved in a patient's care requests a *clinical ethics consultation* concerning a treatment decision. This consultation service may be provided by a clinical ethicist who is employed by an academic medical center, a large hospital, or a health care system, or by a clinical ethicist who works as a consultant, or by a clinical ethics consultation team or ethics committee that includes clinicians and other staff members. Some health care networks employ clinical ethicists who are responsible for developing policy, processes, and training for ethics consultation teams throughout the organization, and for consulting on complex cases as needed.

At many institutions, however, ethics consultations are conducted by staff members with little or no formal training in ethics and whose expertise and processes are unclear. Variation in how ethics consultation teams approach similar cases at the same institution and across institutions with similar demographics is a recognized problem. Clinical ethicists with advanced academic training and significant experience in ethics consultation are working to develop national consensus on training and credentialing in this specialized area of bioethics.[36]

An institution's ethics program is likely to include an *ethics committee* as a forum to discuss and learn from difficult cases and to develop recommendations concerning policy and processes in order to address frequently arising ethical problems in patient care. The membership of the ethics committee may include or overlap with, but is usually not identical to, that of the ethics consultation team. Some larger institutions may have specialized ethics committees for pediatrics or other patient subpopulations raising special concerns. At some institutions, the ethics committee is not yet a robust service that is well integrated into clinical care, with a recognized value to clinical staff. Instead, it may function merely as a crisis committee, a grievance committee, a risk management committee, or a committee of last resort.

In the United States, clinical ethics programs are usually associated with hospitals and with the decisions about life-sustaining treatment and care near the end of life that take place in ICUs, other inpatient settings, or the emergency department. While ethical challenges involving decisions about life-sustaining treatment and care near the end of life also arise in nursing homes and home care agencies, these institutions may lack an infrastructure (including grand rounds and other educational opportunities familiar to hospital-based clinicians) that regularly raises awareness of these challenges and how to respond to them. This can make it difficult for nursing homes and home care agencies to sustain an ethics committee, with a diverse membership, whose mission and value are clear to all staff.

In addition to providing ethics consultation and an ethics committee, an institution needs to provide *ethics education*. This is best understood both as formal education and a continuous, institutionally supported process of ethical reflection and discussion. A strong ethics education program within an institution also encourages clinicians to take part in external programs, such as palliative care training, that can further support good practice. However, as with ethics consultations and ethics committees, there is significant variation in the quality of ethics education and how much institutions are willing to invest in developing an ethically competent professional staff.

As treatment decisions about life-sustaining treatment and end-of-life care routinely raise ethical questions, institutions that provide care to seriously ill patients should:

### 1. Establish a strong and competent ethics program

All institutions that provide care for patients who face decisions about life-sustaining treatment or are nearing the end of life should recognize the need for a structure to identify, discuss, and resolve ethics problems associated with treatment decision-making. Institutional leadership and the leadership of the ethics program should avoid confusing the function of this program with that of risk management. While ethics services may contribute to the resolution of conflicts and problems that could give rise to claims, the patient-centered goals of an ethics program may sometimes conflict with the institution-centered goals of risk management.

### 2. Establish policy and processes for ethics consultations

An institution's policy concerning its ethics consultation service should reflect an understanding of the situations in which ethical concerns over treatment decision-making and patient care arise in that care setting. This policy should reflect familiarity with model processes for conducting ethics consultations. Some institutions use a single model for all consultations, while others use different models for different types of consultations. Any ethics consultation process and policy should offer a reliable, systematic structure for what is necessarily a fluid process. The institution's policy and processes for ethics consultations should cover:

- the goals of ethics consultation;
- who is accountable for the functioning of the ethics consultation service;
- who is qualified to perform ethics consultation;
- who can request an ethics consultation;
- examples of requests that are appropriate for ethics consultation, how to make these requests, and who must be notified at the time of a request;
- examples of requests that are not appropriate for ethics consultation and where such requests should be directed;
- the ethics consultation model(s) used by the institution;
- how the confidentiality of participants in an ethics consultation will be protected;
- how an ethics consultation will be performed;
- how an ethics consultation will be documented; and
- how the quality of the ethics consultation service will be assessed and assured over time.

For resources on ethics consultation, see the Bibliography supporting this section, and also the web-based resources included in the Bibliography.

### 3. Establish policy and processes for ethics committees

An institution's policy concerning its ethics committee should support an effective structure for retrospective learning from past cases, for prospective discussion of ethical issues arising in care delivery, and for identifying and responding to ethics education needs within the institution. To be effective, an ethics committee should have:

- adequate staffing, including, at minimum, a chairperson who has training or other experience in health care ethics, who can effectively lead small-group work, and who is respected within the institution;
- a clear mission, a clear process for educating staff about its mission and how to make use of its services, and the resources necessary to allow the committee to fulfill its mission;
- accountability to the institution's top leadership, including a mechanism for reporting to leadership;
- processes for recruiting and training new members and for the continuing education of all members;
- a diverse membership reflecting the diversity of the patient population, professions, and staff in the institution;
- transparent systems, including processes for scheduling, announcing, and conducting meetings, for note-taking and distributing meeting notes within the committee, and for protecting the confidentiality of written and oral communications; and
- methods for evaluating and improving the quality of the services it provides over time.

### 4. Establish expectations and support processes for ethics education

An institution's policy should address the role of the ethics committee in leading ethics education within the institution. The institution's staff should be able to rely on the ethics committee to offer them substantive opportunities to learn about and reflect on the ethical dimensions of clinical practice. Because other clinical and administrative departments and services (including the institution's office of legal counsel) may also offer educational programs for clinicians that are relevant to ethical practice, the scope of ethics education in an institution is likely to include collaboration with departments and services beyond the ethics service. Ethics education that is accessible to physicians in community practice and to health care professionals in other institutions who care for patients facing decisions about life-sustaining treatment or nearing the end of life may help to strengthen ethical practice and improve care throughout a community.

As discussed in the guidelines on the role of institutional legal counsel and risk management in supporting good care (see Part Two, Section 6F, below), educational collaboration among an institution's ethics service, legal counsel, and risk management department may be especially important in correcting misinformation about the law as it applies to patients facing decisions about life-sustaining treatment and patients who are near the end of life.

### 5. Create and review policies and procedures specific to decisions about life-sustaining treatment and care near the end of life

An institution's policy should address the role of the ethics committee in developing and periodically reviewing the institution's policies and procedures. An institution's leadership, including its trustees, should be able to refer policy questions to the ethics committee for discussion and to receive timely and well-informed recommendations on these questions. Policies should address treatment decision-making, including how to conduct clinical evaluations to determine decision-making capacity, and how to proceed when a patient without decision-making capacity lacks a surrogate. This guidance should include:

- a written procedure for how decision-making about life-sustaining treatment should proceed when a patient lacks decision-making capacity and has no surrogate, including referral procedures for ethics consultation; and
- education and training for members of ethics consultation teams concerning the patient without decision-making capacity who lacks a surrogate, including situations in which it may be necessary to seek a court-appointed guardian.

These *Guidelines* propose nine ethics competencies (see Part One, Section 2) for professionals who care for patients who face decisions about life-sustaining treatment and patients nearing the end of life. They further recommend that institutional leaders support the practice of ethically competent care by establishing these competencies as educational expectations and by investing in education to help professionals to develop these ethical competencies. The Bibliography cites extensive research and other resources supporting these competencies.

## B. Guidelines on Palliative Care Services

These Guidelines recommend the integration of palliative care—including management of pain and symptoms and access to supportive services such as mental health care, professional chaplaincy, and social work—into treatment and care plans in all care settings for all patients, including patients near the end of life. This integration should begin upon admission through upfront screening for palliative care needs and should be maintained through all care transitions. This is an ethical imperative for health care institutions and an ethics education priority. Palliative care services should also encompass the support of loved ones involved in the care of dying patients and address their grief and bereavement.

Palliative care is an interdisciplinary specialty that involves physicians, nurses, mental health professionals, social workers, chaplains, and other professionals. There are models for delivering palliative care in hospitals and nursing homes, through home care agencies and other outpatient settings, and through hospices that deliver pre-hospice palliative care and the well-established hospice model. Materials on these models are now readily available, as are standards for assessing the quality of an institution's palliative care services. The web-based research and educational resources included in the Bibliography feature many tools for developing, assessing, and improving palliative care services.

The integration of pain and symptom management into care near the end of life in U.S. health care institutions is a work in progress. The benefits of the full integration of palliative care into health care from diagnosis onward are quantifiable for patients and for institutions. However, some professionals may still incorrectly associate palliative care solely with situations in which therapeutic interventions have ceased. They may be unsure when to call for a palliative care consultation or how to collaborate with specialists in palliative medicine and nursing. Palliative care services may not be fully reimbursable and may require institutional investment.

All health care institutions should integrate pain and symptom management into patient care. Health care institutions that care for persons near the end of life must do so.

As seriously ill patients are likely to experience pain and symptoms and have other palliative care needs, institutions that provide care to seriously ill patients should:

1. **Invest in palliative care services appropriate for the needs of their patient population**
An institution should identify palliative care models appropriate for their patient population and care setting. Necessary investments may include training for all clinical staff in the fundamentals of palliative medicine, the recruitment of a team of palliative care specialists, and collaboration between institutions, such as a hospice program and a nursing home.

2. **Regularly review and improve existing institutional processes by which professionals, patients, and loved ones gain access to pain and symptom management services, including but not limited to palliative care consultations**
An institution should seek to learn how its palliative care service is perceived by professionals and other staff in all patient care settings within the institution, including those that provide care to patients facing decisions about life-sustaining treatment or who are near the end of life. These settings include ICUs and medical and surgical units serving adult and pediatric patients, the emergency department, and also outpatient facilities for patients undergoing dialysis, chemotherapy, and other life-sustaining treatments. Learning about clinical perceptions of palliative care and how accessible an institution's palliative care services are to patients in different care settings helps identify any structural barriers to

access. Coupling quality improvement measures with palliative care education and training opportunities may increase knowledge of pain and symptom management and encourage a shared vision of good care.

### 3.  Use system-generated data to identify gaps in access to palliative care

Systemic approaches to improving palliative care use data to identify patients diagnosed with conditions indicating an ongoing need for palliative care in order to train the professionals responsible for these patients' care to assess and address palliative care needs. Data suggesting gaps in access to palliative care provide evidence that institutions should review their performance in palliative care and check for discrepancies in access across groups.

### 4.  Ensure that access to palliative care is maintained during care transitions

Ensuring access to palliative care is particularly important during transitions, including transfers of responsibility for patient care between professionals (hand-offs). Shift changes should include a review of each patient's pain, symptoms, medications, and other palliative care needs and the completion or updating of any medical orders prior to a hand-off to incoming staff.

Transfers between care settings should include a review of palliative care needs and the completion or updating of any medical orders and prescriptions that will accompany the patient to his or her destination prior to initiating transfer. Transfers between care settings (including between a medical unit and a hospice unit in the same facility) should include contact between the responsible professional in the patient's current care setting and the professional who will be responsible for palliative care at the patient's destination to ensure that all ordered medications will be available at the destination. In particular, the discharging health care professional should ensure that the patient is provided with an adequate supply of all necessary medications and with prescriptions and other documentation required to support the safe and effective use of all prescribed medications.

### 5.  Establish policies and processes to assure access to mental health services, social services, and chaplaincy for patients and loved ones when decisions about life-sustaining treatment and end-of-life care are being made

Clinical practice guidelines for palliative care encourage institutions to recognize the interdisciplinary nature of palliative care and to involve specialties beyond medicine and nursing in providing it. An institution's policy and processes should support access to mental health services, spiritual care services, and social services for patients facing decisions to forgo life-sustaining treatment and patients approaching the end of life, and for surrogates and loved ones involved in a patient's care. The integration of screening tools into admission processes and other interviews with patients can help ensure this access by eliciting patient concerns and promoting referrals as needed. For example, a "spiritual screen" is a short set of questions designed to help physicians and nurses quickly identify and make referrals for patients whose suffering may have a spiritual or religious dimension that a board-certified chaplain may be able to address if desired by the patient.[37] By providing the responsible professional with a way to elicit more information about the patient's concerns, the planned use of screening tools can also facilitate communication between the responsible professional and other team members who may be able to provide support during decision-making and end-of-life care.

For descriptions of screening tools used to identify palliative care needs, see the Bibliography supporting this section, and also the web-based resources.

**6. Promote collaboration among palliative care providers across care settings**

Patients forgoing life-sustaining treatment or nearing the end of life may need to receive palliative care as they move across settings that include hospitals, hospices, and nursing homes and other types of long-term care facilities, as well as home. Hospital-based palliative care professionals may be best situated to promote ongoing collaboration among professionals and staff who are involved in the delivery of palliative care in a community with the goal of identifying common concerns, developing knowledge and skills, and improving care and continuity of care across settings. Opportunities for collaboration may include ethics education, interdisciplinary grand rounds and other continuing education programs, and projects to explore ways for professionals at different institutions to work together.

## C. Guidelines Supporting Advance Care Planning

As described in Part Two, Section 1, advance care planning is a process for discussing and documenting a patient's preferences concerning the goals of care and the care plan that best achieves these goals. Advance care planning helps to achieve the ethics goals that inform these *Guidelines*, including patient self-determination concerning treatment decisions and how patients wish to live out their lives as individuals and as participants in social relationships.

This process may include the completion of written advance directives, including treatment directives and the appointment of a health proxy, to guide treatment decision-making in the event that the patient loses decision-making capacity. When patients do not complete an advance directive or proxy appointment document, advance care planning may involve other documentation of patient preferences in the medical record. Health care institutions should support advance care planning through policy and processes that help professionals conduct such planning with patients and ensure that the documents and records created through advance care planning will be used in patient care. Institutional advance care planning processes should include attention to the educational needs of professionals, patients, surrogates, and loved ones. Because advance care planning involves documentation that may be relied on by different professionals at different points in a patient's care, the "system"-level guidelines presented here are crucial to the ability of individual professionals to follow the "bedside"-level guidelines in Part Two, Section 1.

The sheer number of professionals involved in the care of a seriously ill patient over time means that advance care planning should be an institutional priority. The care of hospitalized Medicare-eligible patients often depends on a rotating set of staff hospitalists. Although the use of hospitalists can improve continuity of care by ensuring that a particular physician on each shift has responsibility for each patient's care, shift changes may introduce discontinuity and create safety hazards by interrupting the flow of information among members of a health care team. ICU personnel and other critical care specialists who may be responsible for the care of patients facing decisions about life-sustaining treatments or nearing the end of life also rotate frequently. Operational systems should protect patients from being harmed by discontinuities. Advance care planning and the staff training and information technologies that support it should be recognized as crucial to patient safety.

Institutions that provide care to patients with chronic, progressive, or life-threatening conditions should:

1. **Establish policy and processes for advance care planning**

This policy should describe the ethical importance of offering advance care planning to patients, developing a care plan that reflects patient preferences, and monitoring and improving advance care planning processes to ensure that patients' rights are protected and their preferences are honored. Such a policy is in keeping with the federal Patient Self-Determination Act. The policy should clarify that advance care planning can be completed with or without written advance directives. It should neither pressure patients to complete written advance directives nor penalize patients who choose not to do so. Processes supporting this policy should include:

- a process for screening patients to determine whether they want to complete written advance directives and for supporting completion of advance directives if desired by the patient;
- a process for documenting a proxy appointment or other designated surrogate for every patient who has completed a proxy appointment or designated a surrogate;
- a process for documenting treatment preferences for every patient who has completed a treatment directive;
- a process for developing a care plan, including how to elicit patient preferences, identify the goals of care, and formulate and document a care plan, whether or not a patient has completed written advance directives;
- a process for regularly reviewing existing treatment directives, including any documents that may have originated in a different care setting, to ensure that they accurately reflect the preferences of the patient;
- a process for ensuring that advance directives and documentation of patient preferences in the patient's medical record are available across care settings;

- a process for regularly reviewing the patient's goals of care, including documented preferences about treatment options and care settings, and for ensuring that the care plan reflects the patient's goals;
- a process for identifying any preferences and goals that should be written as medical orders (the use of portable medical orders [see D, below] that consolidate any existing advance directives is also recommended);
- clinician education in advance care planning processes and the use of care plans; and
- access to ethics consultation services as needed to support advance care planning.

2. **Collect data on advance care planning processes and outcomes and use data to improve both and ensure equitable access**

Systematic data collection can aid in understanding how well advance care planning is working across an institution or health care system. This analysis can also help determine whether there are gaps in access to advance care planning that need to be addressed.

## D. Guidelines Supporting Portable Medical Orders

Institutional policy should support the ability of physicians and other health care professionals to work with portable medical orders for the care of patients who may face foreseeable medical emergencies. Institutions in states or communities with a program modeled on the POLST Paradigm (see Part Two, Section 4) should ensure that institutional policy supports the use of the standardized document created through a POLST-type process to safeguard the rights and honor the decisions of patients who have completed this process, as well as the decisions of their surrogates. For the same reason, institutions in states or communities that have not yet authorized a POLST Paradigm program should ensure that institutional policy supports the use of other types of portable medical orders. In the interest of equity, institutions should strive to offer all seriously ill patients access to a POLST-type process.

Institutions that provide care to patients who have portable medical orders or may find them useful should educate patient care staff in the preparation and use of these documents, with attention to:

- state law and policy supporting the use of portable medical orders, including POLST-type processes, with examples of any standardized form authorized for use in a community or state;
- how portable medical orders are used across care settings and jurisdictions;
- how portable medical orders concerning foreseeable medical emergencies arising from serious illness relate to treatment directives prepared in advance by patients. For example, portable medical orders are created in direct consultation with a physician,

while advance treatment directives often are not. Portable medical orders offer specific guidance concerning contingencies and are authorized for use by emergency medical personnel and other health care professionals who may not have ready access to other information, such as advance directives.

- how to create portable medical orders as part of advance care planning involving seriously ill patients facing foreseeable medical emergencies;
- how to create portable medical orders as part of discharge planning;
- reviewing portable medical orders at a patient's destination and converting or integrating them into standing medical orders in this setting;
- reviewing and updating portable medical orders in response to a patient's changing condition; and
- educating patients, surrogates, team members, hospital emergency department professionals and staff, and community medical personnel in the use of portable medical orders.

# E. Guidelines Supporting Care Transitions

As described in Part Two, Section 4, transfers of responsibility for a patient's care occur from one professional to another within a care setting ("hand-offs"), and also from one care setting to another, as when a patient is transferred from a nursing home to a hospital or discharged from a hospital. Given the frequency of such transitions in health care and the potential harm that discontinuities in care pose to seriously ill patients, health care institutions should recognize good hand-offs and transfers as integral to good practice and should have policy and procedures to support care transitions. This includes policy and processes that support professionals' ability to execute safe transfers of responsibility within a care setting and whenever a patient is moved, transported, or discharged. It also includes policy and processes that provide for the accurate and consistent transfer of patient information, including documents related to advance care planning, between professionals and across care settings that may use different information technologies or rely on different combinations of electronic and paper documentation.

Institutions that provide care to seriously ill patients should:

1. **Establish policy and processes that support good hand-offs within and good transfers across care settings**

Policy should identify good hand-offs and transfers as a moral mandate for all health care institutions in order to provide safe and effective care that reflects treatment preferences. Processes for transfers of responsibility for the care of a seriously ill patient should ensure that:

- the patient, loved ones, and team members receive the name and contact information for the professional who currently has overall responsibility for a patient's care (the "responsible professional"), as well as for any other professionals who may be responsible for this patient's medical and nursing care during the current shift;

- during hand-offs, the professional receiving responsibility for a patient's care during the next shift (or other staff rotation) is made familiar with the most recent clinical evaluation of the patient's decision-making capacity, knows the name of the patient's proxy (if any) or other surrogate, and knows the status of any pending or foreseeable treatment decision that may cross into the next shift;
- the professional receiving responsibility for a patient's care during the next shift is made familiar with any foreseeable medical or nonmedical problems that should be monitored during this professional's shift;
- the professional receiving responsibility for a patient's care during the next shift is made familiar with the patient's documented goals of care, including treatment decisions reflected in these goals and relevant medical orders, and will document any changes to the patient's care plan, or to the goals of care, that may occur during this professional's shift; and
- any team member who observes a change in the patient's condition can communicate this rapidly to the professional responsible for care during the shift for prompt action. This action may require consultation with the professional with overall responsibility for this patient's care.

Processes for transfers of responsibility when discharging a patient or moving the patient to a new care setting should ensure document portability across care settings that may have different information technologies. The use of portable medical orders is recommended for documenting any standing orders and related advance directives. The use of a distinctive and recognizable form for other medical information that should travel with patients during transfer and discharge, including documentation of current medications and allergies, pending lab work, and the name and contact information of the patient's outpatient physician (if different from the responsible professional) is also recommended.

## 2. Address unresolved ethics and/or communication issues related to care transitions

Institutional policy and processes should clarify how professionals and other staff involved in care transitions can resolve or manage care problems prior to hand-off or transfer. These problems may include interpersonal conflict or uncertainty about how decisions concerning life-sustaining treatment or care near the end of life will be made in the new care setting. Policy and processes should include access to ethics consultation, as this may be needed prior to transfer from a hospital to a nursing home or other setting to address a care problem, particularly if ethics consultation is not available at the patient's destination.

3. **Collect data to identify outcomes of care transitions and have a process for improving practice**

Data collection and analysis can pinpoint opportunities and focus strategies for improvement, including better training of professionals and teams, more effective use of available electronic and nonelectronic resources, and better collaboration among institutions. An institution's ethics service and its patient safety or quality improvement department can collaborate to identify opportunities to improve transfers of responsibility for the care of patients facing decisions about life-sustaining treatment or near the end of life. Whenever possible, efforts to improve transfers should involve staff in all institutions that are regularly involved in care transitions for such patients, including hospitals, nursing homes, home care agencies, and hospice programs.

## F. Guidelines on the Role of Institutional Legal Counsel and Risk Management in Supporting Good Care

A health care institution's legal counsel may include one or more staff lawyers, outside counsel, or a combination of these. An institution's risk management department, whether or not it is formally part of the institution's legal department, may work closely with legal counsel. Myths about the law concerning decisions about life-sustaining treatment and care near the end of life tend to reflect professional and institutional fears about legal risk. The guidelines that follow may help health care risk managers and legal counsel dispel these myths and support good care.

Institutional legal counsel and risk managers have an ethical responsibility to support the goals of health care, including care for patients facing decisions about life-sustaining treatment or nearing the end of life. By virtue of their professional knowledge, counsel and risk managers have a special role in improving such care. They should welcome opportunities to collaborate with an institution's ethics program in ethics education and in policy development.

Institutional legal counsel and risk managers should:

1. **Have up-to-date knowledge of federal and state law and regulations relevant to treatment decision-making and care near the end of life**

Clinicians who provide care for patients facing decisions about life-sustaining treatment or nearing the end of life are responsible for knowing relevant federal law and the law of the state in which they practice. Legal counsel and risk managers should support clinicians' ability to learn about and comply with relevant law and to be aware of any special provisions that may affect the delivery of care in a particular state or care setting. Legal counsel and risk managers can accomplish this by maintaining their own professional knowledge of current law, legal and policy trends, and customary practices in the industry, and by sharing their expertise through regular participation in ethics education. The Cited Legal Authorities lists references relevant to the legal, regulatory, and public policy framework of these *Guidelines*. The Bibliography includes citations to the health law literature relevant to the ethical framework of these *Guidelines*.

### 2.  Recognize legal uncertainty

Legal counsel should recognize that questions concerning treatment decision-making in individual cases may involve areas in which the law is ambiguous, only partially developed, or silent. In areas of uncertainty, legal counsel may nonetheless be asked to offer guidance and counsel. Explaining where the law gives clear guidance and on what issues uncertainty prevails is part of educating health professionals.

### 3.  Correct legal misunderstandings

Misperceptions about the law, including myths about legal liability associated with treatment decision-making and care near the end of life, can compromise patient care. These misperceptions may circulate at all levels of an institution, with the potential to affect clinical practice and administrative processes. By virtue of their professional knowledge, legal counsel and risk managers have an obligation to distinguish myths about the law from current law and policy, and they should be able to recognize and correct these misunderstandings. Imparting accurate information about the law on end-of-life care should be a priority in ethics education and in counseling by lawyers and risk managers.

### 4.  Differentiate risk management from ethics consultation

Ethics is not synonymous with law. Institutional policy and processes should recognize that the mission of the ethics committee and the goal of ethics consultations is not to reduce institutional risk through the prevention of claims. While institutional legal counsel and risk managers may serve on the ethics committee, their presence and participation should not govern the committee's priorities and activities. Similarly, an institution's ethics consultation team should have working relationships with, but be independent of, the institution's legal and risk management departments.

## G. Guidelines on Conflict Resolution

Conflicts over treatment decision-making and care near the end of life may be complex, involving relationship and communications issues as well as ethics. The interpersonal conflict itself—whether it arises among a patient's loved ones, among members of a health care team, or between loved ones and a team—may be the reason that someone calls for an ethics consultation. Prolonged hospitalization or frequent readmission of a patient in deteriorating health, a continually changing health care team, and loved ones experiencing fatigue and distress all can lead to miscommunication and mistrust. Differing opinions among team members about a patient's prognosis or care plan can also lead to disagreements; these may be fueled by long-standing tensions between professions or specialties. Team members may also avoid interactions with patients or loved ones who are perceived as difficult. In all of these situations, the ethics consultation team or another trusted professional in an institution may be called on to resolve the conflict.

The goals and techniques of conflict resolution are different from the goals and techniques of ethics consultation. Patients, loved ones, and health care teams may benefit from access to both of these services.

**Institutions that provide care for patients facing decisions about life-sustaining treatment or nearing the end of life should establish policy and processes for conflict resolution in the health care setting.**

An institution's policy and processes for conflict resolution should reflect an understanding of the situations in which conflicts arise in that care setting. They should reflect familiarity with current models for resolving conflicts. At least one such model (bioethics mediation) has been developed specifically for use in health care settings.[38]

Institutional policy should cover:

- the goals of conflict resolution for conflicts over treatment decision-making and patient care;
- who is accountable for the institution's conflict resolution processes;
- who can request conflict resolution services;
- who is qualified to resolve conflicts and how qualified staff are trained and deployed;
- how the confidentiality of parties involved in a conflict resolution will be protected, including protection from any punitive action;
- how conflict resolution will be performed;
- how a conflict resolution attempt, whether successful or unsuccessful, will be documented; and
- how the quality of the institution's conflict resolution processes will be assessed and assured over time.

**Health care institutions have an obligation to inform patients, surrogates, health care professionals, and other health care institutions in advance about any institutional policy restricting treatment options or treatment decisions. If patients or surrogates request treatment options inconsistent with such policy, the institution should cooperate in a patient transfer. If transfer is not possible, the institution should seek to respect patient or surrogate choices.**

Some health care institutions have formal commitments to religious or other principles. These may prompt the institution to object to certain treatment decisions by a patient or surrogate. Institutions should consult legal counsel on the rules applicable to this situation.

Institutions that do not provide certain treatments or that restrict patients' options to forgo treatment should notify patients and surrogates of this as early as possible, preferably before admission and in writing. Institutions' policies limiting treatment choices should also be publicly posted, preferably on the institutional website where they can be seen by prospective as well as current patients. Physicians and institutions that may refer patients to this institution should be notified of the policy as well.

An institution should cooperate in transferring a patient to a different institution if the patient or surrogate wishes to make a treatment choice not allowed at this institution. However, transfers may not always be possible. In such cases, the institution should avoid harm to the patient and seek to respect patient or surrogate choices. It may be necessary to seek judicial resolution.

For guidance concerning conscientious objection by individual professionals, see Part Two, Section 2I ("Conflicts and Challenges Related to Treatment Decision-Making").

# PART THREE

---

# Communication Supporting Decision-Making and Care

# Communication with Patients, Surrogates, and Loved Ones

## The Ethical Importance of Communication and Collaboration in End-of-Life Care

Good care for patients facing decisions about life-sustaining treatment or nearing the end of life involves communication and collaboration with the patient and, unless that person objects, with loved ones involved in the patient's care, including but not limited to the patient's surrogate. Some health care settings, such as hospice, are designed to support family caregivers and other loved ones as well as patients. Other care settings vary in the resources—staff, services, amenities, physical space—designated for this kind of support. Within a single institution, attention given to this aspect of care may vary by the culture and resources of a particular unit or by the presence or absence of role models demonstrating good practice. Implementing the ethics competencies summarized in Part One, Section 2, of these *Guidelines* can promote consistency across settings in which loved ones are involved in caregiving.

This section supports the decision-making guidelines for adults in Part Two, Section 2, by describing effective communication in situations that clinicians who care for seriously ill patients will encounter regularly. The pediatric decision-making guidelines in Part Two, Section 3, include detailed descriptions of communication and collaboration in pediatric care settings.

This section of Part Three also supports the three sections that follow, which discuss specific aspects of communication:

- Part Three, Section 2, discusses communication about life-sustaining treatment with patients who live with different types of disabilities.
- Part Three, Section 3, discusses the psychological factors that professionals are likely to encounter in decision-making about life-sustaining treatment and in end-of-life care.

- Part Three, Section 4, discusses communication about different types of life-sustaining treatments and about other decisions for seriously ill patients and those near the end of life.

Part Three, Section 5, is a discussion guide for institutions that supports communication on resource allocation and the cost of care when patients or surrogates face decisions about life-sustaining treatment or care near the end of life.

## A. Conducting a Family Conference When a Patient's Condition Is Deteriorating

Professionals responsible for the care of seriously ill patients should expect that they will regularly need to help patients, surrogates, and loved ones understand and adjust to changes in a patient's condition and prognosis.[39] The term "family conference" is frequently used to describe a discussion about prognosis, goals of care, and treatment decisions when this discussion is convened by clinicians and includes not only the patient, but also the patient's surrogate (if any) and other loved ones, unless the patient objects. On occasion, it may be necessary to convene a family conference swiftly in response to an emergent situation.

As described below, the family conference can be used recurrently as a forum to support the processes of care planning and decision-making for seriously ill patients, as described in Part Two, Sections 1 and 2. (The collaborative process described in Part Two, Section 3, shows how family conferences can be integrated into family-centered care for children of different ages.)

The catalyst for convening a family conference is often a deterioration in the condition of a patient who may or may not still have decision-making capacity. If the patient still has decision-making capacity, including the patient in any family conference that is expected to produce decisions about care is essential. However, a patient with decision-making capacity has the right to exclude loved ones from the discussion of his or her care and so may insist on an individual conference instead of one with family. Even when a patient lacks decision-making capacity, the patient may be able and willing to participate in this discussion and may help guide surrogate decision-making.

A family conference can be extremely useful when decisions about life-sustaining treatment or care near the end of life need to be made. The conference offers an opportunity for clinicians to provide support to decision-makers and loved ones who are facing potentially difficult decisions and the prospect of the patient's death. All professionals who are responsible for the care of patients facing decisions about life-sustaining treatment or nearing the end of life should know how to plan, conduct, and follow up on family conferences. Professionals who care for patients in critical-care settings may need guidance and education on how to convene and facilitate family conferences that may involve discussion of complicated diagnoses, technologies, and medical information, with involvement of different specialists. Training clinicians to conduct family conferences well should be a priority in ethics education for physicians and nurses.

Before a family conference, the responsible professional together with the other members of the patient care team should:

- Review what is known about the patient's diagnosis, prognosis, current condition, and treatment options and fill in any gaps in the clinicians' understanding. This may include consultation with the patient's community-based health care providers.
- Review what is known about the patient's social circumstances and the loved ones involved in this patient's care, including how any prior decision-making by or on behalf of this patient has taken place. For example, a member of the health care team, such as a physician, nurse, social worker, or chaplain, may have noticed whether the patient's surrogate receives support from other loved ones, or whether loved ones have conflicting perceptions about a patient's preferences and what constitutes acceptable quality of life for this patient. A surrogate may have spoken to a team member about the stress of decision-making. A team member may know whether the patient or loved ones have talked openly about treatment choices and the possibility of the patient's death. Sharing this information within the team prepares the responsible professional and other team members to communicate effectively during the family conference.
- If the patient has decision-making capacity, seek his or her permission to include others in the care conference and ask the patient which loved ones (or others) should be included. Encourage the patient to allow inclusion of any individual he or she has designated to serve as surrogate or who is otherwise likely to serve as surrogate if the patient loses decision-making capacity in the future.
- Whether or not the patient has decision-making capacity, communicate with the patient and loved ones concerning the reason for the conference and who will be participating, as well as specifics, such as time, location, agenda, and privacy protections.
- Address any disagreements among members of the health care team or consulting specialists concerning diagnosis, prognosis, treatment options, and the likely outcomes of these options, in view of the patient's current condition.
- Determine which clinician will lead and which other professionals will participate in the family conference. Clinicians who will participate in the conference should also prepare psychologically by acknowledging their own emotional responses to the patient and loved ones and to the patient's health circumstances. Some clinicians may also hold beliefs concerning the quality of life of persons living with certain disabilities. Because these beliefs could unduly influence how this clinician assesses and presents the potential benefits and burdens of life-sustaining treatment when a disabled person is seriously ill, these beliefs should be acknowledged and discussed prior to the conference.

During a family conference, the responsible professional should:

- Introduce everyone present.
- Describe the goals of this conference.

- Find out what the patient (if participating) as well as the surrogate (if any) and other loved ones understand about the patient's situation. Responses to a question such as, "What is your understanding of where things stand now?" can identify medical information to be updated, terminology to be clarified, or unexpressed beliefs about the patient's diagnosis, prognosis, condition, and treatment options. When following up on responses to this question, clinicians should:
  - Avoid jargon and euphemisms, as they may be misunderstood.
  - Avoid using test results or other technical information as a substitute for explaining prognosis. Characterizing a test result as "good" or "stable" when a patient's overall condition is deteriorating is confusing and can be misleading.
  - Correct factual errors and outdated information, mindful that the history of a patient's illness and treatment may include details known to the patient and loved ones but not to the clinicians currently responsible for a patient's care.
- Review what has happened and what is happening to the patient. Describe the patient's prognosis clearly, acknowledging uncertainty while clarifying the likely course and what options and outcomes are no longer possible in view of the patient's condition. Review the patient's current palliative care plan and clarify the kinds of care the patient will receive no matter what is decided concerning life-sustaining treatment.
- If the patient no longer has decision-making capacity, frame the decision at hand in terms of "What would the patient want?" If necessary, remind the surrogate and others present that the standards for surrogate decision-making must be the basis for answering this question. (See Part Two, Section 2D, "Surrogate Decision-Making.") This means that the answer should be based on the patient's explicit preferences concerning treatment or, if those do not exist, the surrogate's assessment of what the patient would want based on knowledge of and experience with the patient. If the surrogate cannot infer the patient's preferences and values, the surrogate should decide based on what would be in the patient's best interests. Use repetition to confirm that participating clinicians have an accurate understanding of the surrogate's decision. Ask the patient (if able to participate) as well as the surrogate and other loved ones if they have any concerns related to this decision.
- If life-sustaining treatments will be withheld or withdrawn and the patient's death is expected to follow, discuss what the patient's process of dying is likely to be like, when death is expected to occur, and how and where continuing palliative and nursing care will be provided to the patient.
- Acknowledge emotions and tolerate silence.

At the conclusion of a family conference, clinicians should:

- Confirm that there is shared understanding of the disease and treatment issues discussed.
- Confirm how the patient's treatment and care will now proceed, including supportive care offered to loved ones.

- Ask if the patient (if able to participate), surrogate, or loved ones have any questions, and let them know which clinician they can contact to answer questions as they may arise. Providing contact information in written form, such as business cards with names and phone numbers, is helpful to the patient, surrogates, and loved ones as a memory aid and so they can direct questions to appropriate staff.
- Write appropriate medical orders to put the decisions into effect.

## B. Supporting the Decision-Maker When Loved Ones Disagree

Professionals caring for patients facing decisions about life-sustaining treatment or care near the end of life sometimes express concern when a loved one previously unknown to them—such as an adult son or daughter who does not live nearby—arrives on the scene and challenges the decision of a patient or a surrogate. The newly arrived loved one may stand in a close biological or social relationship to the patient or surrogate. Professionals should be prepared to orient the newly arrived loved one and help integrate this individual into the decision-making process already under way.

As the responsible professional's first obligation is always to the patient, this professional must focus on caring for the patient and collaborating with the person who has decision-making authority concerning this patient's treatment, whether the decision-maker is the patient or surrogate. This may require the responsible professional to talk privately with the decision-maker to review the patient's prognosis and clarify the goals of care. For example, the responsible professional or another member of the health care team may be concerned that a patient with decision-making capacity, or a patient's surrogate, will have difficulty following the patient's own preferences in the presence of other loved ones, or the responsible professional or another team member may observe that a patient's or a surrogate's decision changes suddenly following the arrival of a loved one.

In such cases, the responsible professional should talk privately with the patient if the patient has decision-making capacity or is able to express preferences, and also with the surrogate if the patient lacks decision-making capacity. Conferring privately may help the responsible professional to determine whether the patient or surrogate is experiencing undue pressure to choose a particular treatment option or to change a decision. It also may help to ensure that a patient or surrogate understands the consequences of a decision that will alter the goals of care and the care plan. Another member of the team, such as a social worker or chaplain, may be able to help support a loved one who has newly arrived and who now seeks to become involved in treatment decision-making.

If a surrogate appears to be placing the interests of others ahead of the patient's wishes and interests (for example, by deciding to continue burdensome treatment because a loved one cannot bear to acknowledge that the patient is dying), or a loved one is unable to support a patient's preferences and so is disrupting care consistent with these preferences, ethics consultation or conflict resolution may be necessary.

## C. Discussing Values Concerning Nutrition and Hydration

This subsection discusses communication about nutrition and hydration, including artificial nutrition and hydration (ANH, also known as "medically provided nutrition and hydration"), when a patient is facing a decision about this form of life-sustaining treatment or is nearing the end of life. These issues may arise during a family conference, as described in subsection A, above.

Ethical and practical issues in decision-making about ANH as a life-sustaining medical intervention that patients or surrogates may choose to forgo are discussed in Part Three, Section 4. Forgoing ANH in the context of advanced dementia is discussed in Part Two, Section 4B ("Care Transitions for Nursing Home Residents").

A patient's surrogate may be uncertain about what should be done when a dying patient consumes very little food or ceases eating and drinking. The surrogate may be distressed by the very prospect of making a decision about ANH. These situations can be a source of disagreement among a patient's loved ones, especially when the patient is a child or adolescent, and may also lead to conflict between loved ones and patient care staff.

A family conference with the responsible professional and other members of the health care team, including a social worker or chaplain, may be helpful in clarifying the patient's overall plan of care and the options for meeting the nutritional and comfort care needs of the patient within that plan. The conference may also develop agreement on the ethically appropriate course of treatment in the context of good care near the end of life. Many dying patients have reduced needs for nutrition and hydration, and a decrease in a patient's desire to eat and to drink is often part of the dying process. Some dying patients may continue to enjoy eating certain foods or small amounts of food. However, forcing nutrition and hydration may greatly burden the dying patient at a time when eating and drinking less may feel more comfortable.

For some patients, ANH presents more burdens than benefits. Explaining to the patient or surrogate and to other loved ones how the patient's comfort will be maintained if the patient or surrogate has decided to forgo ANH is crucial. It is important to address any fears that a dying patient who is no longer eating or who is eating very little food is "starving," or that forgoing efforts to feed the patient constitutes neglect. Airing these fears can help to refocus decision-making and caregiving on the current needs and preferences of this patient. The responsible professional and health care team should clarify that meeting the needs of a patient who is forgoing ANH, or who is dying, may be very different from meeting the nutritional needs of other patients.

Religious teachings on ANH may inform the policies of health care institutions that have specific religious commitments. Any such policies should clarify the ethical and legal rights of patients and surrogates concerning decisions to forgo life-sustaining treatment, including ANH. As discussed in Part Two, Section 6G ("Guidelines on Conflict Resolution"), institutional policies should also provide for the advance notice to patients, surrogates, professionals, and other health care institutions concerning any institutional restrictions on treatment options or decisions. Institutional policies should include a procedure for transfer to another care setting in cases in which a patient's preference or surrogate's decision about ANH (or any other treatment) cannot be honored within the institution and should address how a patient's preference or surrogate's decision will be respected if transfer is not possible.

Religious teachings on ANH may also inform the decision-making of some patients and surrogates. (Some religious traditions may offer more than one perspective on this treatment or may not address it explicitly.) Poorly informed decision-making can result from situations in which patients or surrogates misunderstand the teachings of their own religion or the requirements of the law concerning ANH and health care professionals either fail to address these misperceptions or are uninformed and so cannot clarify matters. The involvement of a knowledgeable board-certified chaplain can help patients and surrogates clarify current religious teachings that may inform their decision-making. The Bibliography for this section includes references that address religious perspectives on these issues. For related guidance, see Part Three, Section 3F ("Religious Objections During Treatment Decision-Making").

## D. Using Electronic and Telephone Communications with Seriously Ill Patients or with Surrogates and Loved Ones

A patient's deteriorating condition may require a responsible professional to work with a surrogate by phone. Whenever possible, it is preferable for the responsible professional and the decision-maker to meet in person for deliberations concerning life-sustaining treatment and the care of a patient nearing death to ensure clear communication.

Seriously ill patients who are receiving treatment as outpatients and loved ones involved in their care may be accustomed to communicating with physicians, nurses, social workers, and other health care professionals by phone or electronically. These methods are convenient for routine communications about ongoing treatment and care. They can improve a patient's access to desired care by enabling a patient to consult with a social worker or receive counseling by phone if it is difficult for a patient to travel, or if these services are not available in the facility where the patient is receiving medical treatment. Professionals responsible for the care of seriously ill outpatients should ask patients and surrogates how they would prefer to be in contact for routine communications. Professionals should also identify any privacy, confidentiality, or other concerns (such as the times of day when patients are best able to participate) related to phone and electronic communications with the patient and with the patient's surrogate and loved ones.

The wide use of phone and electronic communications require professionals to consider the types of discussions that are best conducted in person, even if this is less convenient for patients, surrogates, and other loved ones. Decisions about the goals of care, life-sustaining treatments, or palliative care are important decisions. They should take place in an environment in which there are limited distractions and appropriate attention to privacy and to the psychological support of participants. Whenever possible, the responsible professional should consider traveling to the patient's location to meet, rather than insisting that a seriously ill patient travel to meet with the professional.

---

# Communication and Collaboration with Patients with Disabilities

## Life-Sustaining Treatments and Patients with Disabilities

Patients live with an enormous range of disabilities. Many patients have lived with their disability for a long time and may know more about it, and about their own life with a disability, than health care professionals know. A professional working with any patient who lives with a disability will need to assess his or her own knowledge of the patient's particular disability. The professional should consider whether he or she holds beliefs or stereotypes concerning this disability or the experience of living with a disability that may interfere with good care. If the patient is seriously ill or facing a decision about forgoing treatment that is sustaining life by compensating for a disability, the professional will also need to understand that patients have the ethical and legal right to refuse life-sustaining treatment, whether or not they are terminally ill. (See Introduction.)

The diagnosis of a life-threatening condition in a person who lives with a disability, or the progression of an existing condition, may bring this person into new care settings where knowledge of this person's disability and how he or she is living with it is limited or nonexistent. Clinician education concerning the medical care of seriously ill persons with disabilities should recognize the likely need for collaboration among professionals across care settings. These settings may include acute care hospitals, rehabilitation hospitals, psychiatric hospitals and units, nursing homes and other long-term care facilities, ambulatory care settings, home care, and hospice.

To promote collaborative learning and improve continuity of care, clinician educators in institutions that care for seriously ill patients should seek to involve experts in disability in education for medical and nursing staff. Within institutions, opportunities for ethics education and ethical reflection should address disability-related issues that professionals can expect to encounter. For example, staff at an acute care hospital located near a residential care facility for persons with disabilities may provide medical care to these community residents when needed.

This section discusses several scenarios in which a patient's disability may be relevant to communications with health care professionals, the evaluation of decision-making capacity, or the process of decision-making. This section also addresses communication and collaboration with patients who are making initial decisions about their use of life-sustaining technology in the context of recent disability.

## A. Life-Sustaining Treatments and Accommodation of Stable or Progressive Disabilities

The medical situation of a person with a relatively stable or slowly progressing disability who uses a life-sustaining technology such as a ventilator is different from that of a person with an inexorably progressing disease for whom life-sustaining interventions may have some potential to prolong life but can no longer control the underlying disease process and deterioration. While their medical situations differ, each of these individuals has an ethical and legal right to make informed choices concerning the use of life-sustaining treatment. Neither of them is obligated to use life-sustaining treatment simply because such treatment exists and may be of benefit. Indeed, two different individuals with the same stable or slowly progressing condition—or the same inexorably progressing condition—may reach different decisions about the use of life-sustaining treatment in the context of their own lives and goals.

When a person has a diagnosis of terminal illness, decisions about life-sustaining treatments and technologies tend to be framed as "end-of-life" decisions. When a person does not have a diagnosis of terminal illness but relies on a treatment or technology to replace or significantly supplement a physiological function necessary for life, the decision is somewhat different. A decision to forgo a life-sustaining intervention may mean the person is likely to die as a result, but a decision to continue may mean that the person could live a long time with the support of that intervention. However, the mere fact that continuation of life-sustaining treatment may extend life significantly does not obligate the person to choose that treatment. This means that "chronic," "clinic," or "rehabilitation" settings in which persons with stable or progressive disabilities may receive health care should be recognized by professionals and institutions as settings in which end-of-life decisions may be considered and in which decision-making processes should be supported through education and policy.

## B. Communication When a Patient's Disability Affects Speech

A patient who cannot speak (and who does not use American Sign Language [ASL] or another sign language) may be able to communicate nonverbally, through sounds, facial expressions, gestures, or other voluntary and purposeful physical movement, or through the use of technology, such as an alphabet board or a computer. A speech-language pathologist may help in setting up and facilitating communication with a patient who does not speak or sign. Others who may be able to assist the responsible professional may include a loved one or a primary care provider with knowledge of this patient, or a rehabilitation specialist, psychologist, or social worker with knowledge of this patient's disability. A patient who uses ASL or another sign language should have access to the services of a certified health care interpreter.

Situations that may require ethics consultation include those in which the decision-making capacity of a patient who cannot speak or sign cannot be reliably determined even after clinical evaluation involving a speech-language pathologist. Ethics consultation may also be required when the responsible professional is no longer able to communicate reliably with a patient who may have exercised decision-making capacity in the past. Collaborative decision-making involving both the patient and a loved one or surrogate may provide the process needed to afford these patients the same rights as other patients and to avoid harms resulting from delays in making decisions and providing care.

Some patients with advanced dementia or other forms of cognitive impairment may communicate preferences and reactions nonverbally, through sounds, facial expressions, gestures, and other physical movement. These patients may respond to nonverbal communication, such as touch, eye contact, tone of voice, sound, and facial expression, more readily than they respond to speech. The use of primary nursing and other consistent staff assignment can support communication with a nonverbal and cognitively impaired patient by helping staff to become familiar with how this patient communicates and what forms of communication this patient appears to understand.

## C. Communication When a Patient's Disability Affects Cognition

Cognitive disability may be lifelong or of acute onset, and may be either familiar to the patient or recent and less familiar. Some cognitive disabilities will render a patient incapable of making treatment decisions, while others will not. Some adults with lifelong cognitive disabilities may never have had decision-making capacity and thus will need surrogates for medical decision-making. However, adults with lifelong cognitive disabilities vary enormously in their functional capacities and in how they communicate, and also in their medical needs. Some will be capable of participating in collaborative decision-making with a surrogate and medical professionals and should have the opportunity to do so, as they are willing and able. Others may have limited or no apparent understanding of their medical condition or of the consequences of treatment decisions but may be able to express wishes and preferences concerning their lives, or these preferences may be evident to caregivers. Surrogate decision-making concerning a person with a cognitive disability must always consider how this person may experience and express pain and suffering, including suffering resulting from the inability to continue activities that give meaning and pleasure.

Adults with cognitive disabilities resulting from traumatic brain injury (TBI) or who have psychiatric conditions interfering with cognition may have had decision-making capacity prior to injury or the onset of mental illness. Depending on the nature and severity of their cognitive impairment, some may have the ability to make medical decisions under certain conditions. For example, a patient who lacks decision-making capacity during episodes when thinking is highly disordered may regain decision-making capacity when these symptoms are under control. Some patients with brain injuries may have difficulty understanding information presented in one form but may be able to understand the same information presented in another form.

The clinical evaluation of the decision-making capacity of an adult with cognitive disabilities resulting from traumatic brain injury should include consultation with specialists in the care of patients with brain injuries. For similar reasons, the clinical evaluation of the decision-making capacity of an adult with a known or suspected psychiatric condition affecting cognition should include a psychiatric consultation. In each case, the consultant can perform an evaluation and offer guidance to the responsible professional concerning communication with the patient, collaborative decision-making, and any special surrogacy arrangements that may be needed or appropriate for this patient. Whenever possible, the responsible professional should collaborate with professionals who have been regularly involved in the patient's medical care and whom this patient may already trust.

Managing the medical care of a seriously ill, cognitively-impaired adult may be challenging for medical professionals who are unfamiliar with forms of cognitive impairment other than dementia or who have not participated in medical decision-making involving surrogates who are not family members or other loved ones. For example, a professional responsible for the health care of a patient with a disability affecting cognition who has been diagnosed with a life-threatening but treatable condition may know that this patient has a legal guardian with authority to make medical decisions. However, the professional may not yet know how to work with this type of surrogate. The professional may also be uncertain whether the patient's daily caregivers will be able to manage the ongoing medical needs of a patient who may not understand why he or she is undergoing this treatment and experiencing treatment-related side effects. The professional may want more information about how the burdens of treatment (including restraints, if found necessary to provide treatment) have been or are likely to be experienced by this patient. The patient's experience of burden may lead the professional to question the appropriateness of imposing that treatment. The professional may need ethics consultation and access to palliative care specialists that include professionals with knowledge of this patient's disability. The professional may also need guidance on relevant law and policy to support collaboration with the patient's guardian and primary care providers.

## D. Communication and Collaboration with Recently Disabled Patients Concerning Life-Sustaining Treatments

When a person first sustains an injury (such as some spinal cord injuries) resulting in disability that includes loss or impairment of physiological function needed to sustain life, the life-saving treatment this person receives may include the introduction of technology (such as mechanical ventilation) to replace or supplement physiological function. The person may (or may not) express a belief that "living like this" will be intolerable. The person may also express a desire to have the life-sustaining technology withdrawn immediately. Addressing these concerns requires prompt discussion and sustained attention.

The responsible professional can support this patient's ability to make an informed decision by suggesting a time-limited trial of the technology, as described in Part Two, Section 2E ("Making the Decision at Hand"). It is the patient's choice whether to accept this suggestion. If possible, the patient should be offered opportunities to talk, in person or by other means of communication, with others living with similar disabilities, to find out what the experience of living with this disability is like, whether there is a realistic potential for improvement, and what long-term medical and social supports are available for patients and loved ones adjusting to this disability. These discussions may help inform the patient's treatment decision. The patient should be offered opportunities to meet with rehabilitation medicine professionals. The involvement of mental health professionals and social workers with expertise in working with individuals who have relatively stable disabilities is likely to be helpful to the patient and to the professional responsible for the patient's care.

# Psychological Dimensions of Decision-Making about Life-Sustaining Treatment and Care Near the End of Life

## Introduction

Professionals who care for patients and support surrogates facing decisions about life-sustaining treatment and about care near the end of life should have some knowledge of the ways in which psychological issues can arise in treatment decision-making. This section supports the decision-making guidelines in Part Two, Section 2, by discussing these psychological issues. The Bibliography cites selections from the extensive literature on these issues.

The end of a person's life is often distressing to that person and to those close to them, even when they are receiving good care. It is normal for intense emotions to be experienced by the dying person, by their loved ones, and by health care professionals and paraprofessionals who have become close to this person. The experience of strong emotions—including anger, sadness, regret, joy, anguish, and fear—and of rapid shifts between emotional states, including apathy, can be unsettling. For the patient, some of these emotions may be associated with the presence of pain or other physiological symptoms, or with the alleviation of pain and symptoms. Some emotions may be associated with treatment decision-making, medical crises, grief, or the many questions that the reality of disease progression may raise: Who will raise my children if I am no longer here? Who will finish my life's work if I cannot? Some emotions arise from the psychological complexity of terminal illness in which many days are shaped by the demands of a worsening disease process, awareness of what has been lost, and the loneliness of this experience. Other days may offer pleasure, respite, or the simple freedom to continue to shape one's own life.

The end of life is a psychological experience as well as a physiological experience. Strong emotions and the need to face complex challenges do not necessarily mean that an ethical problem or an interpersonal conflict over treatment decision-making is also present. However, such problems can add to stress when a person is near the end of life.

Clinician education on the psychological dimensions of treatment decision-making and end-of-life care should be available to all professionals and other staff who care for patients who face decisions about life-sustaining treatment and patients near the end of life. This education should include, but not be limited to, members of palliative care and mental health services.

## A. Coping as a Factor in Treatment Decision-Making

When a person is diagnosed with a serious illness or injury, the person and loved ones will initially rely on the coping skills they already have. They may not be sure how to manage the bewildering, at times frightening circumstances in which they now find themselves. Those with prior experience of illness or disability may have already developed ways to cope with the stresses of a life-changing diagnosis, the disruption of routine, and the urgent need to take in new information. Some patients will labor to control intense emotions. Children who are seriously ill may have intense emotions as well as unexpected coping skills. They may even try to protect their parents from the reality of the disease process.

Patients may also have beliefs about how they ought to cope with trouble, perhaps thinking that they should be stoic or should not complain. They may receive contradictory advice on coping from friends, for example, to "never give up hope," but also to "face the facts." Even health care professionals may use contradictory-sounding language among themselves and with seriously ill patients and their loved ones, for example, by continuing to describe the patient as "battling" the disease, even as the patient is accepting his or her condition and preparing to die.

A patient's values and beliefs may be an important part of his or her coping. For some patients, their personal spirituality or their religious beliefs may affect how they cope with illness, by helping them to find meaning in their remaining life and, in some cases, guiding their treatment decisions. Knowing that some patients and surrogates make decisions about life-sustaining interventions with reference to values and beliefs reflected in their preexisting coping practices can be useful to a professional who is preparing to discuss such a decision with a patient or surrogate. The involvement of a social worker or chaplain in this discussion may be helpful in eliciting a fuller understanding of how a patient and loved ones are coping with illness and treatment.

## B. Hope as a Factor in Treatment Decision-Making

A decision to pursue medical treatment in response to the diagnosis of a life-threatening condition is a decision that involves hope: the expectation, under conditions of uncertainty, that there is a real possibility of a good outcome—of getting what you aim for. Hoping is different from imagining, or "wishful thinking." It begins with a realistic understanding of the patient's condition, and then aspires to a good outcome or a positive development, be it an improvement in the patient's overall condition, effective pain relief, or simply a good day. Hoping for a good outcome does not require a person to be an optimist. A person who does not regard himself or herself as a hopeful person, or who thinks of himself or herself as a realist rather than an optimist, can still hope for something he or she values. What a seriously ill patient hopes for is likely to change over time. Early in the illness, the patient may hope for cure. Later, the patient may hope for good quality time with loved ones before life ends.

In communication about treatment options, the responsible professional should clarify what a treatment can and cannot accomplish and the likelihood that it will accomplish its goals so that false hope does not undermine informed decision-making and lead a patient or surrogate to take on burdens they would not otherwise have chosen. It would be unethical for a health care professional to encourage a patient or a surrogate to hope for something that the professional knows is not a possible outcome—for example, that a treatment will cure an incurable condition, or that the use of a symptom-relieving treatment or technology will halt the progression of underlying disease.

The ethics of hope are complicated when a patient or a surrogate is considering an intervention that is certain to be burdensome to the patient but offers some potential for a benefit that is meaningful to them and is consistent with what is known of the patient's explicit preferences or inferred preferences and values. These are difficult decisions, and hope can loom large. A time-limited trial can be helpful in assessing the benefits and burdens of treatment more precisely.

Some health care professionals believe that to "instill hope" is part of their vocation as healers. Some professionals also believe that it is wrong to "take away hope" from their patients. These beliefs can lead professionals to withhold desired information about a poor prognosis or burdensome side effects, although there are no data showing that truthfulness on the part of professionals decreases patients' ability to hope. Rather, research suggests that as an illness progresses, a patient's ability to hope persists, even as the patient is likely to shift from hoping for a cure to hoping for comfort and for connection with loved ones.[40]

The same professionals who value giving hope and supporting a patient's ability to hope may be perplexed if patients or surrogates decide to continue treatment when there is small potential for benefit. These patients and their loved ones may speak of (or be described as) "hoping for a miracle," whether in the form of divine intervention, a low-probability reprieve from disease progression, or a new treatment option. It is hard to draw a sharp line between spiritual or religious and secular ideas about hope in the face of death.

In contemporary American society, choosing to hope can be an expression of self-determination, a demonstration of a person's moral or religious stance, or a way of continuing to participate in a society that values hope. When a person is facing decisions about life-sustaining treatment or care near the end of life, the language of hope can be both comforting and confusing. Hoping for a good outcome from a treatment or the use of a technology can be difficult to sustain when a disease is progressing. For some individuals, simultaneously hoping for the best while bracing for bad news becomes a way of coping with the stresses of illness.

Making a practice of asking, "Can you tell me what you hope for now?" is a way for health care professionals both to acknowledge that the language of hope and act of hoping are important to some patients and their loved ones, and also to clarify what is being hoped for at this point. The patient and loved ones may already have shifted from hoping for cure to hoping for comfort, and it is important for health care professionals to be aware of this. The responsible professional who is presenting treatment options should be prepared to explain whether a hoped-for goal of treatment is not, or is no longer, attainable. The professional should also recognize that hope will continue to be important to some patients and their loved ones even when it is clear that some previous hopes are no longer attainable. As the language of hope can be associated with religious beliefs and practices, the involvement of a chaplain may be helpful in facilitating communication during treatment decision-making and in providing desired support to patients, surrogates, and other loved ones.

Opportunities for ethical reflection and personal reflection offered to professionals caring for persons near the end of life should include attention to the concept and language of hope, including how health care professionals can talk about hope and address their patients' hopes.

## C. Ambivalence, Denial, and Grief as Factors in Treatment Decision-Making

Some patients and surrogates will feel ambivalent about making a decision to withhold or withdraw life-sustaining treatment. Whether or not this patient has previously thought about, discussed, or documented treatment preferences, the patient or surrogate who is asked to make these choices is also being asked to do something difficult: face death. In such a distressing situation, some patients or surrogates may try to sustain what is familiar. Some may avoid making the decision or downplay and even reject evidence that the patient's condition is deteriorating.

Acknowledging ambivalence about decision-making can be challenging for professionals. It is time-consuming to help a patient or surrogate sort out and resolve his or her ambivalence. It is also tempting for professionals to see ambivalence as a denial of reality on the part of the patient or loved ones. However, characterizing a patient, surrogate, or other loved ones as "in denial" can increase tension, impede collaboration, and block adequate support for the patient or surrogate facing distress, grief, and the prospect of loss. Using the processes for family conferences described in Part Three, Section 1 ("Conducting a Family Conference When a Patient's Condition is Deteriorating"), and Part Two, Section 3A ("General Guidelines for Pediatric Decision-Making Concerning the Use of Life-Sustaining Treatments") can help address these situations. The involvement of a team member with expertise in responding to grief may be helpful.

Dealing with ambivalence toward making decisions about life-sustaining treatment and care near the end of life requires professionals to distinguish between an ethically justifiable postponement of the decision for a specified period to resolve the ambivalence and an ethically problematic avoidance of the decision. "Deciding not to decide" while a patient's condition worsens can lead to a drift toward more and more intensive interventions, without clarity as to whether these interventions reflect the patient's explicit or inferred preferences, or are in the patient's best interests. In general, delay is problematic when burdensome to the patient. These situations call for collaborative decision-making involving professionals with strong communications skills and may require ethics consultation.

## D. Existential Suffering as a Factor in Treatment Decision-Making

"Existential suffering" (or "existential distress") is a term used by some health care professionals to describe a patient's subjective sense of suffering in their current circumstances. While there is no consensus definition of this term, it usually refers to suffering that is not relieved by the treatment of physiological symptoms or that occurs in the absence of such symptoms. It can be experienced by religious or nonreligious persons and should not be equated with religious or spiritual distress (described in the subsection that follows) unless described by the person in those terms. For a dying person, sources of existential suffering may include the prospect of death, fear of pain or a health crisis near death, alienation, profound loneliness, and loss of meaning.

When a professional caring for a patient near the end of life finds that this person is experiencing existential suffering, the professional must address this suffering. A psychiatric consultation can help determine if depression, anxiety, or another treatable condition (for example, insomnia) is in fact contributing to the patient's suffering, and to what extent this suffering can be alleviated therapeutically. This consultation may also identify modifiable environmental factors, such as noise or lack of privacy, that are contributing to this patient's suffering. The use of primary nursing, in which one or more specific nurses are assigned to follow a patient during a hospitalization, may reduce existential suffering by providing this patient with continuity and support in bedside care. Social work, chaplaincy, other clergy, and loved ones may also play a role. Above all, staff must be attentive, caring, and ready to listen to the existentially distressed patient.

The intentional use of sedation to reduce awareness of suffering in a dying patient involves a range of ethical considerations. Part Three, Section 4J ("Palliative Sedation") describes current areas of debate with respect to the use of sedation, including to relieve existential suffering.

## E. Spirituality and Religion as Factors in Treatment Decision-Making

Caring for a patient who is facing decisions about life-sustaining treatment or is nearing the end of life means being attentive to the whole person. This person has an inner life and a social identity and has lived in social contexts involving family, friendships, school, work, and community. Persons who know they are facing the end of life may reflect on the meaning of their life as it has been lived. Some individuals express these concerns in terms of a religious faith that has been challenged or reaffirmed by illness and suffering. Other individuals express these concerns about meaning with reference to spirituality rather than to a faith tradition. Others face the end of life with no reference to religion or spirituality.

A dying person's sense of his or her life's meaning may change as this person faces illness and death. Some individuals may reconsider long-standing values and preferences in light of the actual experience of illness and dying. Some may become interested in long-dormant beliefs or find meaning and comfort in practices that have not been part of their lives to date. Some patients or their loved ones may reject certain religious or other beliefs near the end of life or experience feelings of estrangement or abandonment.

The palliative care plan for a patient who is near the end of life should include ongoing opportunities for this patient and loved ones involved in the patient's care to discuss spiritual, religious, or other personal issues in whatever way the patient wishes to define these issues. Health care professionals vary in their interest in and comfort discussing these issues. One patient may feel most comfortable discussing these concerns with a chaplain, while another may prefer to discuss these concerns with a social worker. Some may prefer to talk to a mental health professional, although some patients may be wary of any suggestion that their concerns indicate a psychological problem. Still others may prefer to talk informally with their loved ones or with physicians or nurses with whom they have developed a bond. Some patients may prefer not to talk about these concerns at all.

Professional (board-certified) chaplains are clinically trained to help seriously ill patients discuss spiritual and religious issues that may be important to a patient, as well as broader issues concerning life's meaning. They can also teach other clinicians how to have these discussions and how to determine when a referral to chaplaincy may be helpful. Chaplains can function as members of health care teams or in consultation with teams and are responsible for meeting any specific religious and related cultural needs of a patient or family. They are often also responsible for teaching clinicians about religious or cultural practices, such as rituals associated with the care of the sick or the dying, that may be familiar and comforting to a particular patient. Social workers and mental health professionals may also have relevant expertise. Professionals should consider how to offer spiritual care to seriously ill patients who seek it but are receiving outpatient treatment or home care, settings in which this type of care may be less accessible than in the inpatient, nursing home, or hospice settings in which most chaplains work.

## F. Religious Objections During Treatment Decision-Making

When a patient, surrogate, or loved one asserts a religious objection to making a decision concerning life-sustaining treatment or to a particular treatment option (such as the refusal of blood or blood products), the responsible professional should ask for more information about the nature of the objection.[41] It may be helpful to involve a chaplain as soon as a religious objection is expressed, as chaplains are familiar with communication and collaboration under these circumstances. An objection framed in religious language should not stop discussion.

Sometimes, the religious objection was not identified earlier in the patient's care, or there is a misunderstanding concerning a question of religious doctrine relevant to a patient's treatment preferences. The use of "spiritual assessment" questions at admission or early in care planning can help prevent this problem by offering patients an opportunity to clarify any religious preferences concerning treatment and care and by ensuring that these preferences are documented. Resources for assessing spiritual needs are included in the Bibliography.

Acceptance that the end of life is near, including a decision to forgo life-sustaining treatment, may challenge the religious faith of some patients or surrogates. The prospect of death can be deeply unsettling. Sometimes, a religious objection indicates that a patient, surrogate, or loved ones feel things are moving too fast. Probing the religious objection to explore underlying feelings of distress may be helpful.

Inviting a patient or surrogate and other loved ones to talk about religious concerns early in the patient's care may avert misunderstanding and conflict later. It also allows health care professionals to learn whether the patient himself or herself holds the same religious beliefs as the surrogate or other loved ones. In the patient's care, it is the patient's beliefs, values, and preferences that govern. If the surrogate or loved ones assert a religious objection to following the patient's wishes, discussion about the importance of following the patient's preferences is in order.

A chaplain can collaborate with the responsible professional to address religious objections arising during treatment decision-making. If the objection reflects an unmet religious need or concern among loved ones, the chaplain can collaborate to provide loved ones with appropriate attention while ensuring that treatment decisions follow the patient's explicit or inferred preferences, or best interests, in keeping with the standards for surrogate decision-making. (See Part Two, Section 2D, "Surrogate Decision-Making.") A chaplain may also be able to collaborate with outside clergy who are trusted by a patient or family but may be unfamiliar with the patient's condition or with end-of-life care. In cases where a religious objection does not reflect an unmet religious need, the chaplain may be able to identify the underlying source of distress or to facilitate dialogue if trust between the responsible professional and loved ones has broken down. Ethics consultation and conflict resolution may be necessary in some cases involving religious objections.

## G. Moral Distress as a Factor in Treatment Decision-Making

"Moral distress" refers to the distress experienced by some health care professionals when they perceive themselves to be participating in actions that they feel are morally wrong, and are unable to do what they believe to be morally right. Moral distress may be associated with situations in which the goals of a patient's care are unclear to some (though not necessarily all) bedside staff. Health care professionals may also experience moral distress when they feel forced to follow policies they perceive to be harmful to patients.

The professional experiencing moral distress may feel a general sense of unease or may feel complicit in wrongdoing. The sensation of moral distress can be visceral: A nurse or physician experiencing moral distress may feel as if he or she is being forced to harm a patient. The memory of unresolved moral distress may continue to shape a clinician's perceptions and actions into the future.

Moral distress is often, but not always, associated with interpersonal conflict. The morally distressed professional may disagree with the judgment of colleagues or with the decisions of a patient or surrogate. A history of tension between members of different professions or medical specialties involved in the care of the same patient over a long period can contribute to moral distress.

A situation producing moral distress may go on for some time before being addressed as a patient care problem. Individual efforts to relieve the sensation of moral distress often include avoiding patient contact, informally trading shifts, or even seeking to have a patient transferred to a different unit. These efforts are unsatisfactory ways to manage this problem, as they introduce discontinuities into patient care and do not address whether there is, in fact, something inappropriate about the care the patient is receiving.

Some professionals may consider asserting a conscientious objection to continued involvement in the patient's care or the implementation of a certain treatment decision, in order to resolve their moral distress. Other professionals may believe that to withdraw from a morally distressing case would violate their duty of care. There are several problems with using conscientious objection to resolve moral distress. Conscientious objection should be reserved for managing a conflict between a clinician's professional responsibilities and deeply seated religious or other moral commitments that the clinician can describe. Conscientious objection tends to concern specific treatments or care plans that violate these personal commitments. By contrast, the professional experiencing moral distress may actually find it difficult to describe what he or she perceives to be morally wrong about a particular situation, apart from the general unease he or she is experiencing. Also, a clinician should not assert a conscientious objection to providing treatment simply because the clinician disagrees with a treatment decision or plan. Clinicians and patients may hold different values, and patient care should be guided by the patient's preferences and values. In the rare case of a conscientious objection, clinicians should promptly notify the patient or surrogate (if any) and should participate in the orderly transfer of this patient's care to a different clinician. (See Part Two, Section 2I, "Conflicts and Challenges Related to Treatment Decision-Making.") In the more common case of moral distress, ethics consultation and conflict resolution may be useful to the professional and team.

Ethics education for professionals and paraprofessionals may also be helpful in preventing situations that produce moral distress and in clearing up any misperceptions about the ethics of end-of-life care that may lead to moral distress. Ethics education should include opportunities to discuss this problem. Clinicians may or may not be familiar with the term "moral distress" but are likely to recognize the sense of wrongness and powerlessness characteristic of this experience. Scheduling ethics discussions at times convenient for all professionals and paraprofessionals to participate and offering opportunities for all to participate in the analysis of issues in patient care are ways to invite critical reflection and dialogue. Institutional policy development efforts should acknowledge the problem of moral distress and identify nonpunitive ways to respond to this problem.

## H. Integrating Bereavement Care for Loved Ones and Professionals into Care Near the End of Life

Hospice care often addresses bereavement as part of the care of patients and their loved ones from the time of hospice enrollment. Other end-of-life care settings may not offer as much help to loved ones to prepare for the patient's death and the prospect of their own bereavement. Ethics education and ethical reflection in care settings where decisions are made about life-sustaining treatment and end-of-life care should include opportunities for bedside professionals to learn about grief and the complex emotions associated with devastating loss. Education and reflection should also aim to help bedside professionals address their own bereavement needs and psychological responses to difficult or distressing cases.

# Decision-Making Concerning Specific Treatments and Technologies

## A. Forgoing Life-Sustaining Treatments: Ethical and Practical Considerations for Clinicians

Decisions to forgo life-sustaining treatment encompass decisions to refrain from starting a treatment (withholding) and decisions to stop a treatment (withdrawing or discontinuing).[42] As discussed in the Introduction to these *Guidelines*, withholding and withdrawing treatment are morally equivalent. However, patients, surrogates, other loved ones, and patient care staff may experience these decisions differently. Clinicians require training for both withdrawing and withholding life-sustaining treatment, including what steps to take to ensure that, in either case, pain and symptoms are managed. As discussed in this section, the use of sedation to relieve a patient's intractable pain or symptoms also requires clinical training.

When a patient or surrogate is considering whether to start or stop a life-sustaining treatment, the responsible professional should:

- Review any advance care planning the patient or surrogate has completed to date.
- Clarify the goals of the life-sustaining treatment relative to the patient's underlying diagnosis, prognosis, and condition.
- Clarify whether the patient or surrogate chooses to try the treatment for a defined period using a time-limited trial, as described in Part Two, Section 2, before making a decision whether to continue or stop treatment.
- Clarify how the patient will be cared for and how symptoms will be managed to keep the patient comfortable, as the patient starts, continues, or stops treatment.
- Document the patient's or surrogate's decision concerning the treatment at this time. This may involve documenting the decision in the medical record, updating existing care planning documents, and creating or updating portable medical orders for seriously

ill patients who may be transferred between care settings. (See Part Two, Section 1, and Part Two, Section 4C, "Guidelines on Portable Medical Orders.")

When a patient or surrogate decides that a life-sustaining treatment or technology should be withdrawn because it no longer meets the goals of care or is no longer desired by the patient, the responsible professional should carefully manage the withdrawal procedure, assisted by other members of the health care team and additional professionals as needed. This is especially important when withdrawal could cause the patient discomfort or distress, or when death is expected to follow the withdrawal.

When preparing for treatment withdrawal, including when the patient's death is expected to follow, the responsible professional and team should:

- Document the decision and its rationale in the patient's medical records.
- Describe the withdrawal procedure to the patient (if able and willing to receive this information) and to the patient's surrogate (if any) and loved ones, including:
  - what they will see and hear during and after the procedure;
  - what the patient will experience during and after the procedure;
  - how the patient's comfort will be ensured during and after the procedure; and
  - how long the patient is expected to live following the procedure, taking prognostic uncertainty into account.
- Ask about any preferences concerning end-of-life care that have not already been identified, including which loved ones the patient wants to be present for the withdrawal procedure and what types of support may be helpful to the patient and loved ones. For further guidance on support for both during ventilator withdrawal, see subsection C ("Mechanical Ventilation") below.
- Determine when and where the withdrawal procedure will take place and how the patient will be cared for until then. A patient or surrogate may wish to postpone implementing a decision to withdraw life-sustaining treatment for a brief period to allow loved ones to gather at the bedside. If a patient or surrogate requests a long or unspecified delay following such a decision, an ethics consultation may be appropriate to review the decision and identify any unresolved issues.
- Develop a plan for each step of the withdrawal procedure, including potential complications. Ensure that the plan addresses the patient's foreseeable needs for pain medication or sedation. Determine with the patient and surrogate whether the withdrawal procedure should or should not include tapering, which may have advantages and disadvantages (such as prolonging life in an unwanted way). Review the plan with team members and with any specialists who will participate in the procedure.
- Describe how the wishes of a patient who is an organ and tissue donor will be honored in the context of the withdrawal procedure. If the patient is a potential donor, ask the patient or surrogate if he or she would like to discuss the option of organ and tissue

donation with the transplantation team (as the personnel designated to discuss possible donation should be and usually are separate from the personnel managing treatment and the withdrawal of life-sustaining technologies). For additional discussion and resources, see the Bibliography supporting this subsection, and also Part Two, Section 5 ("The Determination of Death: Continuing Ethical Debates").

- Determine whether the patient is in a setting appropriate for carrying out the withdrawal procedure and for providing subsequent care. For example, this may involve moving the patient from the ICU to a quieter and more private space. In some cases, the responsible professional may recommend to the patient or surrogate that the patient be transferred from the hospital to an out-of-hospital setting, such as a hospice facility or a private home, prior to a withdrawal procedure. Any such transfer should be in keeping with the "General Guidelines for Hand-Offs between Professionals and Transfers across Care Settings," as discussed in Part Two, Section 4A of these *Guidelines*. Transfer for the purpose of withdrawing life-sustaining treatment and allowing the patient to die should not be imposed on the patient, especially if the patient or surrogate objects to transfer. Patients have the right to stop life-sustaining treatment in any setting, and hospitals should be fully able to manage the withdrawal process and patient's subsequent care needs.

- Remove any monitoring devices that are superfluous to the procedure and subsequent care.

- Document the withdrawal procedure in the patient's chart.


## B. Brain Injuries and Neurological States

### Communication about brain injuries and neurological states

Understanding brain injuries (resulting from causes such as stroke, oxygen deprivation, trauma, and infection) and making decisions for brain-injured patients present special challenges.[43] How surrogates, other loved ones, and clinicians who do not specialize in neurology understand neurological states may be influenced by how terms such as "coma" or "brain dead" are used in everyday speech, by media coverage of high-profile cases, or by fictional portrayals of film or television characters who wake up from "comas" after years or decades. The responsible professional should anticipate the need to define terms and correct misperceptions when discussing brain injuries and neurological states with patients, surrogates, and other loved ones. Members of the patient care team and staff working in settings where patients with brain injuries are cared for should also make a practice of clear communication and consistent use of up-to-date terminology among themselves. This close attention to communication supports informed decision-making and care planning by helping all understand a patient's diagnosis and reduces the risk of conflict resulting from miscommunication.

When a brain injury (such as a stroke) reflects the progression of an underlying and terminal disease process, it is essential for professionals to present information about the brain injury in the context of the patient's prognosis and overall condition. A dying patient who has a massive stroke or a series of smaller strokes, because this patient is near the end of life, is different from a patient who has had a stroke that is not the result of underlying end-stage disease. Explaining to the patient (if still able to understand and willing to receive the information), surrogate, and loved ones how the stroke fits into the patient's disease course can help make this change in the patient's condition understandable.

As the surrogate for a brain-injured patient may face decisions related to life-sustaining treatments for comorbid conditions, the material in this Section on decisions about other life-sustaining treatments may also be relevant.

### Neurological states: Key definitions

**Coma** is the initial presentation of severe brain injury. The comatose patient is unconscious, and the patient's eyes are closed. Coma is a temporary state usually lasting no more than several weeks. Depending on the nature and severity of the brain injury, a patient in a coma may return to consciousness or may transition to a different neurological state. The prognosis for a comatose patient following oxygen deprivation to the entire brain (anoxia) is graver than for a comatose patient following a traumatic brain injury (TBI).

**Locked-in syndrome or locked-in state (LIS)** is a rare neurological disorder characterized by complete paralysis of all voluntary muscles except for eye movement. Locked-in syndrome may be caused by TBI, by certain neurological or circulatory diseases, or by medication overdose. The patient in LIS is fully awake and aware but cannot speak or move. Diagnosis of locked-in syndrome should include consultation with a speech-language pathologist to determine whether the patient is able to communicate through blinking or other eye movements. Establishing communication is crucial so that this patient is able to communicate with the responsible professional and other members of the health care team as well as loved ones. Communication also allows the patient to consent to or refuse medical treatment. The care of a patient in LIS should include collaboration with psychiatrists and with rehabilitation specialists to ensure that the sources of this patient's suffering, which may include treatable depression, are addressed.

The vegetative state includes both the **persistent vegetative state** and the **permanent vegetative state** . These two states may both be referred to as "PVS," but the two states are distinct and clarity concerning a patient's current diagnosis and prognosis is crucial. To avoid confusion, some neurologists recommend using the term **vegetative state** (VS) for the diagnosis and providing the prognosis (persistent or permanent) separately, based on the nature of the brain injury and the duration of impaired consciousness.

The persistent vegetative state was first described in 1972 as a state of "wakefulness without awareness" in which the eyes are open but there is no awareness of self or others.[44] Patients who are vegetative do not have cognitive, higher-brain functions, but retain only autonomic, lower-brain functions such as brain stem direction of cardiac and respiratory function and sleep-wake cycles. Thus, they have no conscious awareness. A vegetative state is labeled as "persistent" once it lasts more than a month.[45]

When the brain is deprived of oxygen for eight minutes or more, brain tissue dies and the brain cannot recover from the injury. If the brain injury is the result of anoxia due to stroke, cardiac arrest, or another cause, a vegetative state that lasts for three months is considered permanent. A traumatically injured brain has more potential to recover than does an anoxically injured brain, so it takes longer to conclude that a traumatic injury has resulted in a permanent vegetative state. If the brain injury is the result of head trauma, a vegetative state that lasts for twelve months is considered permanent.[46]

Both the persistent and the permanent vegetative states are eyes-open states of unconsciousness. Pointing out that coma is an eyes-closed state of unconsciousness while the vegetative state is an eyes-open state of unconsciousness may help surrogates and other loved ones to understand the difference between a temporary coma and a vegetative state.

The vegetative state defies normal expectations about awareness and consciousness. Usually, when a person's eyes are open, he or she is aware of himself or herself, other people, and the environment. A patient in a vegetative state can look aware, and the body retains startle reflexes in response to stimuli. As a result, loved ones, health care professionals, and paraprofessionals may respond to a vegetative patient as if the patient were aware. They may believe that it is wrong—disrespectful to the patient, or disturbing to others or to themselves—not to do so. Clinicians and staff may be unsure whether they should correct loved ones who attribute responses to a patient that are not possible, given the patient's neurological state. For example, a patient in a permanent vegetative state can no longer smile with intent, although reflexes may make it appear that the patient is doing so. Professional caregivers may believe that there is no harm in encouraging or failing to correct these misperceptions. However, allowing misperceptions of a patient's diagnosis and prognosis to develop can undermine a surrogate's ability to make informed decisions. It can also lead to tension between a surrogate and loved ones who perceive the patient's condition differently.

Because the vegetative state can be visually and psychologically confusing, the use of clear and accurate language when discussing the patient's condition is essential. Professionals and staff should acknowledge that loved ones are seeing a patient who may appear to be interacting with them or expressing emotion, but should remind them of the nature and consequences of the patient's brain injury.

The minimally conscious state (MCS) is a newer clinical designation for severely brain-injured patients whose neural networks retain some potential for awareness.[47] Patients in MCS may outwardly resemble patients in a vegetative state, and they may have been in a persistent vegetative state before entering MCS. Use of clinical bedside exams to measure neural activity in response to verbal stimuli (such as the patient's name or instructions involving memory and visualization) suggests that patients in MCS have some awareness of self and the environment, though awareness may fluctuate in depth and duration. Some patients in MCS say words or phrases or make gestures. It is not clear how much potential a patient in MCS has for cognitive recovery. In rare cases, a patient may emerge from MCS years or decades after a brain injury by regaining the ability to engage with others, albeit inconsistently, and to reestablish functional communication.

Differentiating minimally conscious patients, who have some potential for cognitive recovery, from patients in the permanent vegetative state, who have no potential for cognitive recovery, can be difficult, and diagnostic inaccuracy is common. Once a severely brain-injured patient with a vegetative diagnosis is transferred from a hospital to a long-term care facility, health care professionals should consider the possibility that a patient who was diagnosed as being in a vegetative state may have improved to MCS. Neurological consultation may be necessary to determine a patient's current neurological state.

As MCS is a relatively new diagnostic category and an area of clinical research, there has been some debate about decision-making for patients in this neurological state, compared to patients in PVS. A patient in PVS has persistent or permanent loss of consciousness and therefore can have no awareness of his or her situation. However, a patient in MCS may be minimally conscious of severe impairment. The standards for surrogate decision-making remain the essential guide, with the surrogate deciding in keeping with the patient's explicit preferences, or if these are not known, the patient's inferred preferences and values, or (if even those are unknown) the patient's best interests. Ethics education for professionals and staff who care for brain-injured patients, including patients with little to no potential for cognitive recovery, should include opportunities to discuss and reflect on treatment decision-making.

### Surrogate decision-making following severe brain injury

Severe acquired brain injuries that render a patient unable to make their own decisions necessitate surrogate decision-makers. The surrogate will be guided by the patient's explicit preferences, inferred preferences and values, or best interests in making treatment decisions, in keeping with the standards for surrogate decision-making. To understand the clinical situation, diagnosis, and prognosis, a surrogate may ask whether the patient will survive this immediate crisis. A more complex pair of questions follows: If the patient survives, will the patient recover or be impaired? And if impairment is likely, what will be the nature and extent of this impairment?

In the immediate aftermath of a brain injury, prognostic uncertainty is usually high. This may or may not be relevant to the treatment decision at hand. Most decisions concerning the use of life-sustaining treatment (including decisions about ventilation with intubation or tracheostomy, artificial nutrition and hydration, and surgeries) occur immediately, or within the first few weeks after onset of the brain injury. Decisions made at this time are almost always made with incomplete information. The surrogate should nonetheless strive to decide in keeping with the patient's explicit preferences or (if these are not known) inferred preferences and values or (if even these cannot be ascertained) the patient's best interests, in keeping with the standards for surrogate decision-making. Greater certainty concerning prognosis often requires the passage of time. As noted, it takes three months to be reasonably certain that a patient with an anoxic brain injury is in a permanent vegetative state, and twelve months to be reasonably certain of this diagnosis for a patient with a traumatic brain injury. Thus, it may take months to determine the potential for recovery (if any) and the probable nature of this recovery.

In situations of prognostic uncertainty involving brain injuries, and *in the absence of an underlying disease process that is expected to result in the patient's death no matter what interventions are attempted*, a time-limited trial of life-sustaining treatments and technologies can help clarify the patient's potential to benefit. This may allow the surrogate to make a better-informed decision concerning whether to continue these interventions or to forgo them. However, the surrogate should not authorize a time-limited trial if this would be contrary to the standards for surrogate decision-making, that is, the patient's explicit preferences, inferred preferences and values, or best interests. For guidance on time-limited trials, see Part Two, Sections 2E and 2G ("Making the Decision at Hand" and "Implementing the Decision").

The surrogate with little or no direct knowledge of severe brain injury needs support from health care professionals in answering fundamental questions: Is the patient aware? What is the patient experiencing? Would this particular patient, with his or her values and preferences, want to continue life-sustaining treatment? What supports are available to surrogates and other loved ones who may be integral to a long-term care plan for a brain-injured patient? Collaborative communication is essential and may need to continue over a prolonged period.

## C. Mechanical Ventilation

The word "ventilator" implies a single technology. However, this word is an umbrella term for a range of technologies, from hand-operated bag valve masks to different types of mechanical ventilation, that compensate for the temporary, progressive, or permanent insufficiency of respiratory function. As these *Guidelines* concern decision-making about life-sustaining treatment, this discussion focuses on mechanical ventilation used as a life-sustaining technology by patients with progressive disease or an acute-onset life-threatening condition. In the care of children and adults in this situation, there are two basic types of ventilation used in acute care and some other care settings (neonatal intensive care units include additional types):

- invasive mechanical ventilation involves an endotracheal tube or a tracheostomy, in the case of intubation generally requires sedation, and is often but not always used continuously in the acute care setting.[48]
- noninvasive mechanical ventilation (NIV) usually involves a removable face mask, generally does not require sedation, and is used continuously or only during certain periods, such as during sleep.

A wide range of conditions may involve a decision about whether to use mechanical ventilation. Life-saving efforts for newborns may involve mechanical ventilation.

Declining respiratory function due to the progression of a neurodegenerative disease or a crisis in the trajectory of an acute or progressive disease affecting major organ systems may prompt a decision about ventilation as well. Temporarily or permanently impaired respiratory function following a severe brain injury may call for a decision about ventilation, as may the support of impaired but relatively stable respiratory function following a spinal cord injury. In considering whether a patient wants to accept ventilator support that will be chronic or long-term, there are significant lifestyle issues that must be discussed, such as speech/communication, eating, mobility, and the amount of assistance required (such as with secretion management). These issues may affect where a person can live.

Clarity concerning the reasons for instituting ventilation, the goals of treatment, and the different types of ventilation technologies that may be appropriate for a patient is essential to informed decision-making and good care. A patient's or surrogate's prior knowledge of mechanical ventilation may reflect a different medical context than the situation at hand. Everyday speech, in which different types of ventilators may be referred to generically as "machines," may also influence how some patients and surrogates think about the desirability of mechanical ventilation.

## Invasive mechanical ventilation: Approaching withdrawal and preparing patients and loved ones

Invasive mechanical ventilation is a life-sustaining treatment whose termination requires careful management to avoid patient discomfort. The establishment and use of a withdrawal protocol that involves pain medication and sedation reduces the risk of discomfort and distress for patients and helps to ensure a sound approach to withdrawal by clinicians.

A protocol for the withdrawal of invasive mechanical ventilation should include:

- directions for pain medication and sedation during and after the withdrawal procedure, continuing as long as needed. Increasing preexisting doses of certain medications may be necessary to ensure patient comfort by controlling pain and distress that could result from the withdrawal. As discussed in the Introduction, studies suggest that the use of pain medication and sedation in this way can relieve symptoms and usually does not hasten death.

- advance discussion of whether the patient or surrogate chooses withdrawal by weaning (the gradual discontinuation of mechanical ventilation) in the context of the patient's explicit preferences, inferred preferences and values, or best interests, and the advantages and disadvantages of weaning. The responsible professional should take care to distinguish "weaning" when a patient is dying (sometimes called "terminal weaning") from the gradual discontinuation of mechanical ventilation (for example, during a patient's recovery process from traumatic injury) to permit a patient to breathe unaided.

- a process for determining whether to remove an endotracheal tube after the terminal withdrawal of mechanical ventilation. The professional should assess whether the patient's comfort is better supported by leaving the tube in place or removing it and should describe how the patient's comfort will be ensured. If the tube will be left in place in the interest of patient comfort, loved ones should be told that it will be visible. If the tube will be removed in the interest of patient comfort, loved ones should be told that they may hear the gurgling of secretions as the patient nears death. For further guidance on managing this aspect of withdrawal, see "respiration changes," below.

Some patients will be awake and aware during a withdrawal of mechanical ventilation. Other patients, due to their underlying condition, the sedating effects of medication, or a combination of factors will be less aware or unaware that a withdrawal procedure is taking place.

When describing the withdrawal of mechanical ventilation to a patient or to loved ones, the responsible professional should address the following:

- Prognosis: The responsible professional should clarify whether death is expected following withdrawal of ventilation or the patient is expected to transition to breathing without ventilatory support.
- Timing of death, if expected: The patient, surrogate, and loved ones should be told how the patient will be cared for if death is expected after withdrawal but does not occur rapidly. Most patients will die within twenty-four hours of terminal withdrawal of ventilation, but some may survive for considerably longer.
- Respiration changes: The potential for upper airway noises after a ventilator is withdrawn and the changes in respiration that can occur as a patient is dying should be described to the patient, surrogate, and loved ones, as they may not know what the gurgling of secretions in the airway of a dying person ("death rattle") sounds like. The patient's comfort should be maintained during and following the procedure through use of analgesia and sedation. However, those who are unprepared for this sound may fear that the patient is choking or is gasping in an attempt to communicate a last-minute desire to be reintubated. In describing these respiration changes, clinicians should help the surrogate and loved ones distinguish between the concerns they may have and the patient's capacity to experience distress. Clinicians should reassure the patient's surrogate and loved ones that the decision to be present as the patient dies and to witness terminal respirations after a withdrawal of mechanical ventilation is a personal decision. Those who want to remain with the patient but believe they may be distressed may find they are able to remain if a nurse, chaplain, or other team member can stay with them to offer knowledgeable support.

### Ethical considerations in proposing noninvasive mechanical ventilation as an alternative to invasive mechanical ventilation

For some patients in acute and chronic care settings, different forms of noninvasive mechanical ventilation can be presented as alternatives to invasive mechanical ventilation. When continuing respiratory crises are foreseeable due to a patient's prognosis and condition, the professional responsible for the patient's care should aim to prevent crisis-driven decision-making by helping the patient or surrogate to understand the patient's current options and by identifying which forms of mechanical ventilation may fit with the patient's goals of care.

Ethical concerns arise when a patient whose condition is deteriorating and who has some potential to benefit from noninvasive mechanical ventilation has expressed a wish to forgo the use of a "ventilator" near the end of life.

Some experts argue that it is appropriate to offer this patient a time-limited trial of noninvasive mechanical ventilation to help alleviate respiratory distress and because this patient's goals may include prolonging life under certain circumstances. Moreover, noninvasive mechanical ventilation may help keep the patient more comfortable than other nonmechanical options. Also, because of the common association of the word "ventilator" with "intubation," this patient's wish to avoid a "ventilator" may reflect a more specific wish to avoid invasive mechanical ventilation.

Other experts argue that if a patient who is near the end of life has already decided to forgo mechanical ventilation, it is not appropriate to propose a different form of this technology. Moreover, they suggest that it would be wrong to assume that a patient who had expressed a wish to forgo invasive mechanical ventilation would have wanted noninvasive mechanical ventilation.

A lack of clarity over whether a preference or decision to forgo invasive mechanical ventilation near the end of life also rules out noninvasive mechanical ventilation can lead to confusion. It is important to clarify the patient's preference or the surrogate's decision with regard to both invasive and noninvasive ventilation. There are situations in which a patient who wishes to forgo invasive mechanical ventilation may choose to permit noninvasive mechanical ventilation. These ethical challenges illustrate the importance of advance care planning.

### Mechanical ventilation in the context of the chronic-care management of degenerative conditions

Individuals with degenerative conditions characterized by progressive loss of respiratory function commonly face decisions about beginning to use some type of mechanical ventilation and, once having started, at what point they may wish to forgo further mechanical ventilation. These decisions may be made by a parent or guardian in collaboration with health care professionals when a condition is diagnosed early in a child's life, and or by an older child or adolescent in collaboration with parents or guardians, or as autonomous decisions by an adult patient with decision-making capacity, or by a surrogate for an adult who lacks decision-making capacity. Educating patients and their surrogates about the foresee-able decisions associated with the patient's diagnosis should begin well before the patient needs mechanical ventilation as a life-sustaining measure, if possible. Decision-making processes may include time-limited trials of ventilation technologies with the opportu-nity to revisit decisions. (See Part Two, Sections 2E, 2G, and 2H, "Making the Decision at Hand," "Implementing the Decision," and "Changing Treatment Decisions.") In some cases, a decision may be revisited years after being made. For example, an adolescent or adult patient may want to revisit decisions made by his or her parents when the patient was a child.

Clinicians who regularly care for patients with degenerative conditions involving progressive loss of respiratory function should know how to conduct advance care plan-ning with their patients. At times, these patients may encounter health care professionals who have not cared for patients using mechanical ventilation as a long-term intervention. Advance care planning should anticipate the possibility that, during an emergency, a health care professional will need immediate guidance concerning the patient's explicit prefer-ences regarding mechanical ventilation and the patient's medical condition may prevent the patient from communicating preferences directly. Having a written record of patient preferences and the patient's care plan readily at hand will be important in such situations, and portable medical orders may be helpful. (See Part Two, Section 4C, "Guidelines on Portable Medical Orders.")

## D. Cardiopulmonary Resuscitation and Cardiac Treatments

This subsection is relevant to decision-making about cardiopulmonary resuscitation (CPR) as a potentially life-saving treatment when a patient is near the end of life. It is also relevant to decision-making about pacemakers and other implantable devices used as life-sustaining treatments for different cardiac conditions.

### Cardiopulmonary resuscitation (CPR)

A patient's prognosis after cardiac arrest depends on the patient's overall condition, the underlying cause of the cardiac arrest, and other factors. In some circumstances, cardiopul-monary resuscitation, a term covering a range of interventions aimed at restoring heartbeat and breathing after cardiac arrest, is an effective emergency treatment that can save lives. For example, when a patient experiences cardiac arrest as the result of a myocardial infarc-tion (MI, commonly known as a heart attack), CPR can help maintain the circulation of oxygenated blood throughout the brain and body until heart rhythm can be restored.

However, when a patient whose overall condition is deteriorating suffers cardiac arrest, the likelihood that CPR will meet its immediate goal of restoring heartbeat and breathing is lower, and the patient's prognosis is likely to be poor no matter what inter-ventions are subsequently attempted. There is a large literature on the outcomes of CPR initiated in various settings and different patient subpopulations. Part Two, Section 4B ("Guidelines on Care Transitions for Nursing Home Residents") and the Bibliography supporting that section include guidance and citations reflecting data on CPR outcomes in nursing homes.

Portrayals of CPR in popular media can prompt members of the public—including patients, surrogates, and loved ones—to form a misleading impression of the nature of this treatment and the circumstances under which it is likely or unlikely to achieve its life-saving goal. In-hospital CPR involving advanced cardiac life support (ACLS) can be a highly invasive procedure that a patient may experience as burdensome. As noted, CPR may have a very low likelihood of success when a patient is already frail and debilitated whether CPR is initiated in or out of the hospital. Professionals responsible for advance care planning and for subsequent treatment decision-making should help patients and surrogates understand the likely outcome and the potential for injury if CPR is attempted, given a patient's diagnosis, prognosis, and condition. A decision to forgo CPR may support the goals of a patient who wishes to die at home or who has decided to forgo other life-sustaining treatments.

All health care institutions should have policies about instituting CPR and the option of "do-not-resuscitate" (DNR) orders.[49]

These medical orders implement the patient's or surrogate's advance decision to refuse CPR in the event of cardiopulmonary arrest. Procedures and ethics education supporting these policies should:

- train professionals responsible for the care of seriously ill patients to:
  - discuss the benefits and burdens of CPR with patients and surrogates,
  - document DNR decisions, and
  - include DNR orders in any portable medical orders (see Part Two, Section 4C, "Guidelines on Portable Medical Orders") and to prepare documentation for use at the patient's destination;
- train all patient care staff to recognize DNR orders and the institution's DNR forms and provide opportunities for patient care staff to improve their knowledge of what DNR orders mean and how to implement them;
- ensure that all forms used to document DNR orders explicitly state that a DNR order documents a refusal of CPR;
- accurately reflect law and regulations (if any) governing DNR orders.

Patients with DNR orders may wish to receive treatments, such as surgery, that are consistent with their goals of care. Some desired treatments may involve the administration of anesthesia. The anesthesia care of patients with DNR orders should include preoperative discussion among the responsible professional and other professionals (such as surgeons, anesthesiologists, and nurse-anesthetists) who may become involved in the care of the patient under these conditions, and also between the responsible professional and the patient or surrogate, if any.[50] These discussions should explicitly address the individual patient's goals and preferences, the medically feasible options for honoring these goals and preferences, and the documentation of the preoperative, surgical, and postoperative care plan for anesthesia care. As the result of these discussions, a decision may be made to suspend or modify the DNR order temporarily during the surgical procedure.

Ethics education on DNR orders and circumstances in which they may be temporarily suspended or modified should be offered to all professions potentially involved in the care of these patients.

## Cardiovascular implantable electronic devices (CIEDs)

Professionals who treat patients who use or may potentially use cardiovascular implantable electronic devices (CIEDs) should understand and be prepared to discuss these common devices as life-sustaining technologies that patients may decide to start, discontinue, or refuse. CIEDs are widely used among elderly patients, who may have relied on these devices to maintain cardiac health for many years. As discussed throughout these *Guidelines*, patients have a basic right to be free of unwanted medical treatment, including CIEDs.

A pacemaker is a device that treats arrhythmias by providing the electrical impulse necessary to produce a heartbeat. Some patients use specialized pacemakers for cardiac resynchronization therapy (CRT) to compensate for more extensive damage to heart function. Professionals should present decisions about pacemakers in the context of a patient's diagnosis, prognosis, and overall care plan, rather than discussing a device's benefits and burdens in isolation. The use and deactivation of pacemakers should be addressed in advance care planning and in subsequent discussions about life-sustaining treatment. Clarifying a patient's wishes and preferences about the use of a pacemaker in the context of the patient's overall health and goals can support surrogate decision-making if the patient subsequently loses decision-making capacity.

An implantable cardioverter-defibrillator (ICD) is a more complex technology that monitors for serious tachyarrhythmias and delivers an internal defibrillation shock when needed. ICDs also have pacemaker function. An ICD is used to prevent sudden cardiac death in persons who have survived sudden cardiac death or are at high risk for it. When a patient is dying, the prevention of sudden cardiac death may no longer be consistent with the patient's goals of care, and dying patients who have active ICDs may suffer painful shocks if they experience ventricular arrhythmias as part of the dying process. ICD deactivation should therefore be explicitly addressed in advance care planning and in subsequent discussions about forgoing life-sustaining treatments, including CPR, for when a patient is near the end of life.

All medical professionals who care for patients who are candidates for some type of CIED or who have an activated device should be prepared to:

- discuss device deactivation with patients or surrogates;
- engage in decision-making with patients or surrogates concerning device deactivation in the context of the goals of care and in relation to other treatment decisions;

- address the implications of DNR orders for the use of CIEDs;
- initiate deactivation and documentation procedures in different health care settings, including settings with and without professionals with electrophysiological expertise; and
- address the palliative care needs of patients during and following device deactivation, including situations in which the patient's death is expected to follow soon after the deactivation procedure is completed.

## Mechanical circulatory support

A variety of technologies may be used for mechanical circulatory support in patients with end-stage heart failure (ESHF). These include implantable devices such as a left ventricular assist device (LVAD), right ventricular assist device (RVAD), biventricular assist device (BiVAD), percutaneous ventricular assist device (pVAD, or "Tandem Heart"), and total artificial heart (TAH). Some forms of mechanical circulatory support may be used as "bridge" therapies for patients who are candidates for heart transplantation until a transplant can be performed or who require temporary support during a period of recovery. Some forms of mechanical circulatory support are also used as "destination" therapies for patients who are not candidates for transplantation. Some technologies, such as extracorporeal membrane oxygenation (ECMO), are used in intensive care settings only.

All forms of mechanical circulatory support are life-sustaining technologies that patients may decide to start, stop, or forgo. Medical professionals who care for patients who are potential candidates for some form of mechanical circulatory support but are not transplant-eligible should be prepared to address advance care planning, treatment decision-making, and patient care during and following the implementation of a decision to withhold or withdraw mechanical circulatory support.

As some of these technologies are newer than others, the extent of available professional guidance may vary on ethical questions, such as those that emerge when a bridge therapy begins to be used as a destination therapy or when technologies are used in combination with one another. The substantial ethics literature on the LVAD may be a starting place for clinician education on this and other forms of mechanical circulatory support. (For a selection of this literature, see the Bibliography supporting this section.) Initially developed as a temporary measure to support patients until heart transplant, LVADs are now used as a destination therapy for patients who meet the criteria for New York Heart Association (NYHA) class IV heart failure and who are not candidates for transplantation. Patients who receive LVADs have a longer life expectancy than those whose heart failure is managed medically. However, the use of LVADs as destination therapy is associated with increased risks of strokes, infection, multiple organ failure, and psychological distress.

All professionals who care for patients who are potential candidates for LVADs or other mechanical circulatory support devices should be prepared to address:

- decision-making with patients or surrogates concerning the benefits and burdens of the LVAD (or other mechanical circulatory support device) as destination therapy, including the patient's prognosis with or without this technology, the goals of device implantation, the risks associated with surgical implantation, device maintenance, and the potential impact of this device on a patient's quality of life; and
- withdrawal of the device due to medical complications or a patient's or surrogate's subsequent decision to forgo this treatment. For example, LVAD withdrawal can precipitate the symptoms of heart failure. Decision-making concerning the withdrawal of the LVAD or another mechanical circulatory support device should address symptom relief and other palliative care needs of patients, including when the patient's death is expected to follow.

## E. Dialysis

Hemodialysis is a therapy that compensates for a period of time for the failure of an organ system necessary for life. Patients with chronic kidney failure (commonly known as end-stage renal disease, or ESRD) who receive a kidney transplant live significantly longer than ESRD patients treated with dialysis. If a patient diagnosed with ESRD is potentially a candidate for a kidney transplant, the patient should be evaluated to determine whether he or she is transplantable. If so, the patient or surrogate should be given an explanation of transplantation options, including receiving a kidney from a living donor or being placed on a waiting list to receive a kidney from a deceased donor. The latter option usually involves being treated with dialysis (potentially for several years) while awaiting transplant.

This subsection primarily concerns decisions about dialysis among patients with ESRD who are not awaiting a transplant. A patient in this situation may not be a candidate for transplantation, or the patient or surrogate may have decided to forgo transplantation.

Most ESRD patients who are not candidates for transplantation choose to start dialysis. Patients can also choose a time-limited trial of dialysis or choose to forgo dialysis altogether. Research suggests that initiating dialysis in patients with chronic kidney failure who are seventy-five years of age or older and in poor overall condition may fail to achieve the life-sustaining goal of this treatment, while adding significant treatment-related burdens.[51] Decision-making about dialysis requires clear communication about diagnosis, prognosis, the patient's preferences (including those concerning other forms of life-sustaining treatment), and treatment options, including the option to forgo life-sustaining treatment.

## Decisions concerning dialysis in the context of renal failure

Some patients or their surrogates may decide to refuse or stop dialysis as part of a decision to forgo any further life-sustaining treatment. The decision to forgo dialysis should be documented as described in Part Two, Section 2F ("Documenting the Decision").

If a patient is in renal failure and the patient or surrogate has not yet made a decision to forgo dialysis, the professional responsible for the patient's care should determine if there is any potential for benefit from dialysis relative to the patient's goals of care and given the patient's deteriorating condition. This may require consulting with a nephrologist. If the responsible professional concludes that dialysis is consistent with the goals of care and has some potential for physiological benefit, the professional should present this treatment option to the patient or surrogate. The professional should clarify that performing dialysis when multiple organ systems are beginning to fail will not halt or reverse the progression of the underlying disease process that is causing the patient's vital systems to fail. The professional should specify what physiological benefit dialysis could provide to this patient. Decisions should be documented.

When a patient or surrogate chooses to start a potentially long-term life-sustaining treatment such as dialysis, advance care planning should be completed or the existing care plan reviewed and updated based on the patient's present medical condition and prognosis. Due to the relatively poor health of most dialysis patients, the support of loved ones is often essential to a patient's ability to receive dialysis, as their support includes transportation and assistance on days when the patient is receiving outpatient treatment. Advance care planning for dialysis patients should include involved loved ones, unless the patient objects. An advance care planning process for patients starting dialysis should clarify that a patient can decide to stop dialysis and should include an explanation of the patient's likely course after withdrawal and the palliative care and hospice services that can be provided to the patient.

## Withdrawing dialysis

If the patient has expressed a desire to stop dialysis and has decision-making capacity, or does not have decision-making capacity but is able to express preferences, the responsible professional should ask the patient why the patient wants to stop treatment. If the patient lacks decision-making capacity, a surrogate will make the decision with patient involvement as the patient is able. Dialysis can be exhausting for the patient and disruptive to the lives of the patient and loved ones. These factors may represent burdens that outweigh benefits for a patient, or they may discourage a patient who wishes to continue treatment. If the responsible professional suspects temporary or treatable depression, the professional should discuss the patient's psychological condition with the patient. Involving a social worker or other professional with expertise in the management of dialysis treatment may assist in this evaluation and in obtaining support for the patient as needed. The responsible professional should also consider whether the progression of a comorbid disease or condition now renders continuing dialysis of questionable value. A patient's or surrogate's decision to forgo other life-sustaining treatments may also make dialysis inconsistent with current goals of care.

The documentation and implementation of a decision to withdraw dialysis should include a palliative care plan. Most deaths from chronic kidney failure occur, on average, eight days after stopping dialysis, with patients maintaining consciousness for the first few days.[52] The palliative care plan should therefore address where the patient prefers to spend the last days of life. Most patients who stop dialysis enroll in hospice for end-of-life care, and the palliative care plan should address transition to hospice if that is consistent with patient preferences. The palliative care plan should also anticipate the need for relief of symptoms associated with death from kidney failure and describe how support will be offered to loved ones who will be with the patient and who may be unfamiliar with these symptoms and how they can be relieved.

## F. Nutrition and Hydration

### Nutrition and hydration: General considerations

Among the life-sustaining treatments that patients, surrogates, and caregivers may need to consider starting or stopping are a set of life-sustaining treatments known as **artificial nutrition and hydration (ANH,** also known as medically provided nutrition and hydration). These treatments may include total parenteral nutrition (TPN) delivered intravenously through a central-line catheter; percutaneous endoscopic gastrostomy (PEG), in which nutrients are delivered to the stomach through a tube sutured into the patient's abdomen; jejunostomy (J-tube), in which nutrients are delivered to the small intestine through a tube sutured into the abdomen; hypodermoclysis, in which nutrients are delivered through a subcutaneous needle or port; the use of a nasogastric (NG) tube to deliver nutrients into the digestive tract; and intravenous hydration. Medically provided nutrition is often referred to as a "feeding tube."

Decisions about ANH can be difficult. As discussed in Part Three, Section 1C ("Discussing Values Concerning Nutrition and Hydration"), some patients, surrogates, other loved ones, health care professionals, or other caregivers attach special moral or emotional significance to end-of-life interventions involving nutrition and hydration. These decisions may be especially distressing in pediatric care due to the symbolism of feeding as integral to the care and nurturing of infants and young children, all of whom rely on others to provide them with nutrition and hydration. Health care professionals who are responsible for the care of patients near the end of life should be prepared to address decisions and concerns about ANH. They should be familiar with current research and consensus recommendations concerning the benefits and burdens of ANH in patients who are near the end of life, including alternatives to ANH when a patient is losing the ability to swallow but may still be able to eat with assistance. (See below.) The Bibliography for this subsection includes a selection of this literature. Professionals should be offered opportunities to discuss this literature and to reflect on their own attitudes, beliefs, and values concerning nutrition and hydration near the end of life. These educational opportunities should also be offered to certified nursing assistants and other staff who have hands-on responsibility for patient feeding and comfort.

Professionals and staff should be able to practice in an environment where there is clear and accurate shared knowledge of law and regulations specific to nutrition and hydration decisions when a patient is near the end of life or facing a decision about life-sustaining treatment. For further discussion, see Part Three, Section 1C ("Discussing Values Concerning Nutrition and Hydration").

### Forgoing artificial (medically provided) nutrition and hydration

The right of patients and authority of surrogates to refuse medical treatment includes refusal of ANH. This invasive medical treatment should not be imposed on patients when it conflicts with their wishes. Health care professionals should frame decisions about ANH as they would frame decisions about any other life-sustaining treatment, discussing the evidence concerning the expected benefits and burdens of this treatment for the patient; the patient's diagnosis, prognosis, and current condition; the patient's preferences, if he or she has decision-making capacity; or, if the patient lacks such capacity and a surrogate is deciding, the patient's explicit preferences, inferred preferences and values, or best interests, in keeping with the standards for surrogate decision-making. ANH should not be referred to as the equivalent of "food and water," as a seriously ill patient, including one near the end stage of a terminal disease, may no longer be able to metabolize medically provided nutrients or to take in fluids without discomfort.

A decision to withhold or withdraw ANH should be documented in the patient's medical records, and the patient's care plan should be updated to include ongoing relief of any symptoms, such as dry mouth, related to this decision. Professionals and staff should know how to care for a patient who is forgoing artificial nutrition and hydration, including how to keep this patient comfortable. The process of withdrawing ANH should not cause significant discomfort to a patient. The responsible professional should assure the patient and surrogate (if any), as well as loved ones, that the patient care team can indeed keep the patient comfortable and should describe and document the comfort care plan.

For further discussion of forgoing ANH in the context of sedation to relieve refractory pain or symptoms near death, see the discussion of palliative sedation in Section 4J.

### Decision-making about nutrition and hydration when a patient develops swallowing difficulties

Persons with advanced dementia frequently develop difficulty swallowing food, and decisions about ANH may involve a patient or nursing home resident in the final stage of this disease. While swallowing difficulties are also associated with the progression of other diseases, such as amyotrophic lateral sclerosis (ALS) or head and neck cancers, most of the data on swallowing difficulties when a patient is terminally ill come from patients with advanced dementia in a nursing home.[53]

This research, and the consensus among medical societies and the national Alzheimer's Association, shows that introducing ANH in an effort to prevent malnutrition, weight loss, or aspiration pneumonia when a person with advanced dementia develops swallowing difficulties is more likely to burden than to benefit the person.[54] Tube feeding usually fails to prevent these problems, thereby limiting its benefits. Some of the burdens associated with ANH in this population include the medical-surgical interventions required to place the feeding tube; the potential for infection at an incision site, leading to the possible need for antibiotics and for hospitalization; discomfort experienced from tube feeding; the likelihood that a person with dementia will require physical or chemical restraint to prevent him or her from pulling the tube out; the physiological and social consequences of such restraint; and the loss of the social benefits of hand feeding, if the patient retains some ability to swallow and receives comfort from being fed.

Sometimes a surrogate opts for ANH even when the burdens to the patient seem to outweigh the benefits. If a surrogate is not given information about the burdens and potential harms associated with the introduction of ANH once a patient with advanced dementia develops swallowing difficulties, the surrogate cannot make an informed decision. If a surrogate is not told what can be done for the patient other than ANH once swallowing difficulties arise, the surrogate may conclude that patients who do not receive ANH are not receiving "care." This belief may be shared by some on the patient care staff, who may associate the use of ANH with the prevention of malnutrition and weight loss in healthier patients and fail to differentiate between these patients and the needs of patients who are seriously ill or dying.

Clarifying how a patient with advanced dementia will be cared for following a decision to forgo ANH supports informed surrogate decision-making. It also recognizes that staff members need to understand how to provide good care to this person. As some patients with advanced dementia continue to enjoy the social and sensory dimensions of being hand fed and tasting food, a palliative care plan following a decision to forgo ANH may include "comfort feeding": hand feeding that is experienced as comfort, and that is stopped if the staff member responsible for hand feeding observes that the patient is choking or distressed. A care plan for a patient who is no longer able to swallow or who has lost interest in eating and drinking should include mouth care (such as swabbing the lips and mouth) to relieve symptoms and provide continued social and sensory contact.

For further discussion of forgoing ANH in the context of advanced dementia, see Part Two, Section 4B ("Guidelines on Care Transitions for Nursing Home Residents").

## Cessation of eating and drinking near the end of life: Clinical and ethical considerations

Near the end of life, patients often cease eating and drinking. Sometimes eating, or the sensation of consuming more than a small amount of food or liquid, is unappealing or physically uncomfortable. Some dying patients will refuse offers of food or will push food trays away. The dying person may lose interest in eating and drinking as appetite and sensations associated with hunger and thirst fade, and may be satisfied with ice chips or mouth swabs to relieve dryness.

A dying patient who stops eating and drinking remains a patient who should receive appropriate and desired care. Informing a patient or surrogate that a patient may cease eating and drinking near the end of life and should not be forced to eat involuntarily is helpful but must be supplemented by instruction on how the patient's comfort will be maintained. Professionals responsible for the care of dying patients who have ceased eating and drinking or who are consuming very little food should know how to maintain comfort, develop a care plan for the last days of life, explain the patient's care needs to loved ones, and ensure that the medical record includes clear guidance for staff concerning the care plan, which may change as a patient's needs and preferences change. Clinician education that includes opportunities to learn from and collaborate with hospice professionals and other palliative care specialists can support good practice.

The responsible professional should be prepared for the possibility of disagreement among loved ones concerning the care plan for a patient who is forgoing ANH or has ceased eating and drinking. Ethics consultation or conflict resolution services may be helpful in such cases. For additional guidance on communication, see Part Three, Section 1C ("Discussing Values Concerning Nutrition and Hydration").

The situation of a terminally ill patient who has stopped eating and drinking but whose disease process does not appear to be at its end stage presents a challenging situation for health care professionals. Determining whether this patient's action has a physiological cause such as nausea or reversible loss of appetite, a psychological cause such as reversible depression, or reflects a desire to die should involve a psychiatric consultation and specialists with expert knowledge of this patient's underlying condition. A terminally ill patient who has stopped eating and drinking should not be forced to do so and invasive means of providing ANH should not be instituted over the patient's objection.

Ethics education should address the care of the dying patient who is forgoing ANH or has ceased eating and drinking and should provide opportunities for staff to discuss their own concerns and professional practice.

## G. Chemotherapy and Other Cancer Treatments

This subsection on decision-making about the use of life-sustaining treatment in the context of advanced cancer covers cytotoxic chemotherapy, which aims to intervene in the progression of disease by killing cancer cells, as well as drug therapies (such as hormone therapies and other targeted biological therapies) that aim to interfere with cancer cell growth.[55]

### Cancer treatment and metastatic disease

Treatment options for cancer patients diagnosed with primary or recurrent metastatic disease have expanded in recent decades. Some forms of incurable cancer can now be managed as chronic conditions. Self-administered oral chemotherapy and different types of targeted therapy have reduced treatment burdens for some patients. Palliative care expertise has become more common in cancer centers. Research has now shown that the integration of palliative care into lung cancer treatment from the time a patient is diagnosed with metastatic disease is associated with longer life as well as better quality of life.[56] Other studies of palliative care in the context of cancer treatment consistently show that palliative care is associated with equal or better survival, reduced distress among caregivers, and reduced end-of-life hospitalizations. A selection of these studies is included in the Bibliography supporting this subsection.

Chemotherapy is a common part of the treatment of cancer patients with metastatic disease. Targeted therapies, such as monoclonal antibody drugs that aim to interfere with specific proteins or processes involved in the growth of cancer cells, are also common in the treatment of certain cancers. Depending on the type and stage of the cancer and the patient's condition and responsiveness to treatment, chemotherapy or other cancer drugs may prolong life for a length of time ranging from weeks to months and even to years. The probability that drug therapy will prolong life also varies by type and stage of cancer and by patient.

Studies from the United States and other developed nations over the past thirty years continue to show that many cancer patients will opt for chemotherapy even when it offers a small chance of prolonging life by only a few weeks to a few months, and with the certainty of toxic side effects.[57] This choice may reflect a desire to prolong life or difficulty facing a decision to stop treatment. A cancer patient whose disease is rapidly or inexorably progressing or is becoming increasingly resistant to chemotherapy may have opted for treatments in the past that proved to be life-saving or that resulted in benefits that were worth significant burdens. For a person who has lived with cancer, in some cases for years, choosing to stop efforts to intervene in the disease can be difficult. A decision to opt for chemotherapy with the prospect of only marginal benefit may also reflect a patient's misunderstanding of his or her prognosis or a lack of basic information about likely outcomes with or without treatment. If an oncologist does not tell a patient in such a situation what the likely outcomes are, this patient cannot make a fully informed decision about treatment.

Another reason that cancer patients may opt for burdensome chemotherapy and other treatment near the end of life is that professionals may continue to offer them treatment without raising the question of whether this still makes sense. Professionals who treat patients with advanced cancer grapple with their own uncertainty over the value of continuing chemotherapy. In emotional and practical terms, it may be easier for an oncologist to order another round of the same treatment or to suggest a new drug or enrollment in a research trial, rather than to raise the question of whether chemotherapy is still a useful way of helping the patient. In view of research findings showing that some patients who use less chemotherapy near the end of life may live longer and also have better quality of life, it is crucial for professionals to reflect on this aspect of their own practice.[58] Oncologists and other professionals involved in the treatment of patients with advanced cancer must be prepared to counsel patients and surrogates when further treatment no longer offers prospect of benefit.

Cancer patients with advanced disease may be offered experimental interventions and nonstandard therapies, especially when standard treatments have failed. Most clinical trials involve research on cancer drugs. Novel therapies for treating cancer may include "off-label" uses of approved drugs, as well as drugs not yet approved and available only through clinical trials or compassionate-use applications to a manufacturer. The fact that cancer patients may be offered enrollment in clinical trials raises ethical considerations. A medical oncologist or other professional responsible for the care of a patient with advanced cancer should be prepared to clarify the difference between established therapy and participation in a research protocol and must be careful to explain whether the clinician is also a research investigator involved in that trial. If so, it may be advisable to have another professional speak to the patient about the option of enrolling in the trial, to avoid confusion and so that the patient does not feel pressure to enroll. Novel treatment raises further ethical concerns. The oncologist should describe in what way the treatment under consideration is novel, whether the treatment would be prescribed off-label, explain what that means, and discuss the level of evidence supporting this use in terms of likelihood of benefit to this patient.

### Establishing goals of treatment for advanced cancer

When a patient is diagnosed with metastatic disease or experiences metastatic progression or a metastatic recurrence, the professional responsible for this patient's care (usually a medical oncologist) should clarify the goals of cancer treatment. The goal in some cases may be cure, but in many cases the disease may no longer be curable. Treatment goals may then include slowed disease progression to prolong life, improved functioning, or the relief of pain or symptoms. Treatment goals may also include the resolution or management of a cancer-related problem, such as pleural effusion. The professional responsible for a patient's care should clarify how each proposed intervention, including different chemotherapy agents available for use, serves the overall goals of this patient's care, to ensure that the patient or surrogate can make an informed decision about this intervention.

The institutional process for eliciting and documenting patient preferences concerning cancer treatment and care should promote collaboration among medical oncologists, palliative care specialists, and other professionals involved in the care of a patient with advanced cancer. The documentation of care decisions and goals of care should be accessible whenever professionals involved in inpatient and outpatient care are communicating with one another and with the patient or surrogate.

### Reviewing the goals of treatment when cancer treatment fails

When the responsible professional concludes that a cancer treatment is failing to deliver physiological benefit and that remaining treatment options offer only small potential for marginal benefit, or when the burdens of treatment appear to be outweighing the benefits, the professional should again review the goals of treatment with the patient, or with the patient's surrogate if the patient lacks decision-making capacity. This review supports the patient's ability to plan for the rest of his or her life. A patient or surrogate may sense that treatment is failing and request such a review, which they should be able to do at any time.

In reviewing the goals of treatment and addressing any remaining options for cancer treatment, the professional should clarify:

- the patient's current goals and the patient's current attitude toward continuing treatment;
- treatment options, including the option to forgo further interventions and to shift the focus of care to palliative care or hospice, which may offer a more effective way to meet the patient's goals and to obtain physiological and other benefits;
- whether the professional has a recommendation for the patient or surrogate concerning the value of continuing or discontinuing treatment as a means of achieving the patient's goals;
- the goal of any available treatment in terms of benefit to the patient, such as "less pain" (tumor response by itself may not translate into benefit to the patient);
- the evidence in support of a treatment's ability to provide benefit to the patient, with reference to this patient's history of treatment response and to the data on this treatment;
- whether there is any evidence in support of the treatment's ability to prolong life, and if so, what is known or can be anticipated about the quality of additional life that may be afforded to the patient by this treatment;
- the toxicities and other foreseeable burdens associated with this treatment;
- any out-of-pocket costs associated with this treatment (providing this information helps patients and loved ones to assess cost-related burdens and avoid unanticipated financial stress); see Part One, Section 4B ("Economic Context") and Part Three, Section 5 ("Institutional Discussion Guide on Resource Allocation and the Cost of Care"); and
- whether a time-limited trial of this treatment can be offered and how benefit will be assessed; see Part Two, Sections 2E and 2G ("Making the Decision at Hand" and "Implementing the Decision").

In preparation for this meeting, the responsible professional should identify other professionals who may become more involved in the patient's care if the goals of care shift to palliative care or hospice or if treatment may continue but with a greater role for palliative care. Oncologists in private practice or who work in outpatient settings may have less direct access to professionals with palliative care expertise than oncologists who treat inpatients in cancer centers. However, as oncologists in practice may care for patients with advanced disease, they should be familiar with local services for these patients, including hospice programs and palliative care programs, which may be offered in institutional settings or through home care agencies. Oncologists in practice should also know whether it is possible to offer patients the option of an informational appointment (sometimes called a "pre-referral") with local hospice providers to introduce this service to patients while they are still receiving treatment. Doing so helps patients to understand that hospice care may be part of the effective management of advanced cancer. Pre-referral appointments are usually welcomed by hospice programs as a way to support a patient's ability to plan and to let patients and loved ones know that a transition to hospice can begin well before a patient is near death.

Any decisions made during or following a meeting to review the goals of treatment should be documented. If a patient or surrogate decides to forgo further treatment, the responsible professional should outline the patient's care options going forward. In some hospitals, a patient who is forgoing cancer treatment may have the option of transferring to a palliative care service or hospice program within or affiliated with the same institution. In many situations, a patient will enroll in a hospice program that is separate from the institution in which the patient has been receiving treatment and care. A social worker can assist with these care transitions.

To support continuity of care, the patient's oncologist should continue to be involved in this patient's care after the implementation of a decision to forgo further treatment, if and for as long as this involvement is desired by the patient or surrogate. For example, in the weeks after a patient is referred to hospice, the oncologist can stay in touch with the patient and loved ones through a weekly phone call or other means of communication. This promotes continuity of care, provides the patient or surrogate with an opportunity to ask questions during this transitional period, and communicates the oncologist's continued concern for the patient's well-being during a period of adjustment. For further guidance concerning transfers of responsibility for patient care near the end of life, see Part Two, Section 4 ("Guidelines for Care Transitions").

Ethics education for oncologists and other professionals involved in the care of patients with advanced cancer should aim to promote the integration of palliative care into cancer treatment, in view of the evidence that early and sustained collaboration between oncology and palliative care specialists produces better outcomes for patients and their loved ones. It should also aim to support the ability of oncologists, patients, and surrogates to collaborate in discussion, decision-making, and care planning when cancer treatment may have ceased to provide benefit to a patient, or when treatment burdens are outweighing benefits.

## H. Routine Medications, Antibiotics, and Invasive Procedures

Medications that are commonly administered in health care settings and medical procedures such as blood draws are considered part of "routine medical care." (Antibiotics are separately addressed below.) Because these medications and procedures are so familiar, the question of whether to forgo them may be overlooked during decision-making and care planning near the end of life. The common use of a medication or procedure does not mean it should always be used. When a patient's condition is deteriorating, routine medications and procedures, as well as medications used to treat chronic conditions or acute problems, may cease to benefit this patient and may be experienced as burdens. Patients or their surrogates may refuse medications and invasive procedures, even if these are customarily viewed as "routine." However, some patients who have decided to forgo treatment for a terminal disease process may decide that they wish to receive other medical treatment. For example, a patient who decides to forgo further chemotherapy and who wishes to avoid hospitalization during the remainder of her life may decide to continue to use oral antibiotics to treat minor respiratory infections, in the interest of greater comfort and in an effort to prevent a systemic infection.

The responsible professional should support the patient's or surrogate's ability to make informed decisions by clarifying the benefits and burdens of a medication or procedure in the context of the patient's overall condition and prognosis, rather than focusing on the value of the medication or procedure in isolation. The professional should also clarify whether a decision to forgo a medication or procedure is expected to affect the trajectory of the patient's disease process. Stopping blood draws may have no effect other than to increase comfort, while forgoing medication for a chronic condition or acute problem may shorten the patient's remaining life. The professional should describe how the patient will be cared for if a decision is made to forgo some or all medications and procedures other than those desired by the patient or needed to relieve pain and symptoms. All decisions to forgo medications and procedures should be documented in the patient's medical record. The patient's care plan should be updated to fully anticipate the need for palliative care to provide symptom relief. It is important to clarify in the patient's record what medications and procedures are still accepted by the patient or surrogate to provide palliative care, in order to assure that all members of the patient care team are aware of these decisions.

### Medications for comorbid conditions

Advance care planning, and the ongoing review of a seriously ill patient's care plan to ensure that it reflects the current goals of care, should address a patient's use of medications for chronic comorbid conditions. These medications may include statins, anticoagulants, synthetic thyroid supplements, insulin, steroids, hypertension medications, iron supplements, and many others. These medications may have bothersome side effects, or their continued use may conflict with a patient's or surrogate's decision to forgo life-sustaining treatment. A seriously ill patient may also find certain types of medications, such as pills or injections, burdensome. When a patient or surrogate is making decisions concerning life-sustaining treatment or when a patient's condition is deteriorating, the question of whether to continue these medications should not be overlooked.

### Antibiotics

Antibiotics save lives by treating life-threatening bacterial infections and are given routinely to patients with signs of infection. Health care professionals are well aware of problems associated with the wide use of antibiotics, including the development of antibiotic-resistant strains. However, no contemporary health care professional would want to practice medicine without the option of using antibiotics that can be life-saving or can resolve a biological cause of pain and symptoms. Seriously ill patients who are vulnerable to infection due to a disease process or treatment that affects the body's immune system may take antibiotics regularly.

Patients or surrogates may refuse antibiotics, just as they may refuse other life-sustaining treatments. When a patient's condition is deteriorating due to the progression of underlying disease, the burdens of antibiotics, which can include nausea and other side effects, can outweigh whatever physiological benefits they may achieve. Antibiotics can also cease to be effective when a patient contracts repeated infections as a consequence of deteriorating health, as when a patient who is losing the ability to swallow food repeatedly develops aspiration pneumonia. The use of antibiotics may also conflict with decisions to forgo other forms of life-sustaining treatment. When the responsible professional diagnoses or suspects an infection in a patient who is near the end of life, the professional should evaluate the patient to determine the benefits and burdens of administering antibiotics and discuss this with the patient or surrogate. Precise diagnosis of an infection may appear to require invasive procedures or hospital admission, but if the patient is likely to suffer disproportionately from such measures, professionals should consider whether treatment decisions can be made on the basis of a presumptive diagnosis.

When a hospital patient or nursing home resident is diagnosed with a highly contagious infection, protecting the health and safety of all patients may require professionals to follow public health protocols to prevent or control a disease outbreak. These measures, which are consistent with the ethical goal of equity as described in Part One, Section 1, may compel the professional to consider overriding the patient's refusal of antibiotics and administering antibiotics without consent, or isolating infected patients. Such steps require ethics consultation and may require judicial authorization. In the absence of a clear threat to public health, however, a patient's preferences should prevail.

Some untreated (or treatment-resistant) infections, such as necrotic wounds, may be distressing to members of the patient's health care team, including nurses responsible for wound care, as well as to patients and loved ones. In such cases, an ethics consultation with the team may be helpful to discuss staff distress, ensure that responsibility for this patient's care is distributed equitably among team members, and clarify the right of the patient or surrogate to refuse unwanted treatment.

## Invasive procedures

Care planning, and the ongoing review of a seriously ill patient's care plan, should address invasive procedures commonly associated with hospitalization or with the treatment of a particular disease. These procedures include blood draws, the surgical placement of catheters, and surgeries to resolve acute problems that may be related or unrelated to a patient's underlying disease. Invasive procedures can be uncomfortable, painful, or psychologically challenging for any patient and may be especially burdensome to seriously ill patients. Some diagnostic procedures, such as CT scans and MRIs, can be burdensome as well. Certain invasive and diagnostic procedures also require sedation or anesthesia that may be experienced as a burden by some patients.

Health care professionals can help patients and surrogates address whether any invasive or other burdensome procedures are no longer necessary and desired and so can be withheld or withdrawn. Ethics education in clinical settings should include consideration of procedures that are usually part of routine patient care but that may be unnecessary or unduly burdensome and refused by the patient or surrogate, especially when a patient is near the end of life.

## I. Blood Transfusion and Blood Products

Blood transfusions, like other life-sustaining interventions, may be refused by the patient or surrogate. Refusal of blood and blood products for religious reasons raise special issues, discussed below.

### Decisions concerning the treatment of bleeding associated with progressive disease

Some patients experience hemorrhagic bleeding or anemia due to internal bleeding as a consequence of a progressive disease process, such as cirrhosis of the liver or some cancers. For these patients, blood transfusion may have the potential to sustain life as a stop-gap measure but not to stabilize or reverse a disease trajectory. When bleeding crises are foreseeable, the professional responsible for the patient's care should address the benefits and burdens of blood transfusion with the patient or surrogate, in the context of determining the patient's wishes and preferences concerning life-sustaining treatment and the goals of care. The professional should also clarify what is likely to happen and how the patient will be cared for if the patient or surrogate decides to forgo blood transfusions, and the patient subsequently experiences a life-threatening bleed. If the patient or surrogate decides to forgo blood transfusions, this decision should be documented in the patient's medical records. To provide clear guidance to emergency medical personnel, portable medical orders are recommended as documentation for patients who have decided to forgo blood transfusions and are being transferred or discharged to a different care setting (see Part Two, Section 4C, "Guidelines on Portable Medical Orders").

Situations in which a patient whose condition is deteriorating continues to receive large quantities of whole blood or platelets as a stop-gap measure can raise ethical concerns among medical and nursing professionals. Whole blood and platelets are scarce resources, raising ethical questions if a hospital's blood bank is receiving regular requests on behalf of one patient who can obtain only temporary benefit from this treatment. This resource allocation problem calls for institutional policy. To prevent *ad hoc* bedside rationing, including a blood bank's refusal to supply blood after repeated transfusions, ethics education in institutions caring for critically ill patients should include opportunities to discuss this resource allocation problem and its consequences for patients and clinicians. Part Three, Section 5 ("Institutional Discussion Guide on Resource Allocation and the Cost of Care"), offers models for conducting resource allocation discussions at the institutional level.

Some patients refuse blood transfusions, or all blood products, due to their beliefs about the safety of these products, or for some other reason. In such cases, the responsible professional or another member of the team caring for the patient should seek to ensure that this refusal reflects an informed choice and is not influenced by misinformation about risks associated with blood products. If blood substitutes are appropriate for this patient, the professional should describe this alternative.

## Patients who refuse blood transfusions and blood products for religious reasons

Patients who self-identify as Jehovah's Witnesses may refuse blood transfusions on religious grounds and may also refuse medical treatments involving certain blood products, such as platelets, red cells, white cells, plasma, and cryoprecipitate. Some blood components, such as albumin, immune globulins, and factor concentrate, and blood substitutes may be appropriate for and acceptable to these patients. As each patient is an individual, it is important for the responsible professional to ascertain the patient's actual preferences concerning emergency and other life-sustaining treatment, rather than assuming what those preferences are based on the person's religious affiliation. If the professional becomes concerned that the patient feels pressured to refuse blood or blood products in the presence of loved ones or others, the professional should speak to the patient privately to ascertain his or her transfusion preferences.

To guide professionals in these situations, institutional policy and processes should address blood transfusion and the care of patients who refuse blood and blood products on religious grounds. Institutional policy should emphasize the need to identify and address patient refusals of blood and blood products well before a surgery or an emergency in which transfusion may be indicated. Addressing the refusal in advance will allow discussion with the patient or surrogate of the risks of refusal and alternatives such as blood substitutes. In addition, some surgeons may be more comfortable than others operating while honoring the refusal of blood and blood products on religious grounds; identifying patients who assert such a refusal will allow appropriate planning. When patients refuse blood and blood products on religious grounds, ethics consultation services should be available and should have a process for assisting in these cases. Prompt ethics consultation and legal review are necessary in cases involving minors whose parents or guardians refuse transfusion for them as Jehovah's Witnesses, as parents or guardians are significantly more restricted in their authority to refuse blood or blood products for a minor than for themselves.

Ethics education for clinicians should clarify the rights of patients who refuse blood and blood products and the responsibilities of clinicians caring for these patients. The Bibliography for this section includes a selection of the recent literature on clinical, ethical, and legal considerations in cases involving patients and surrogates who refuse blood or blood products on religious grounds. This literature can aid in education and policy development and support good practice.

## J. Palliative Sedation

In the context of medical care near the end of life, palliative sedation refers to the use of sedating medications to relieve refractory and intolerable symptoms, such as pain, dyspnea, and agitated delirium, after all other measures have failed.[59] (Palliative sedation is usually differentiated from other palliative interventions involving sedating medications, such as time-limited "respite sedation" to relieve and potentially resolve a bothersome symptom such as insomnia.) A reduction in the patient's level of consciousness is anticipated and accepted as a necessary part of this therapy. In palliative sedation, the goal of palliation changes from the control of symptoms in a patient who is fully conscious to a goal based on a joint acceptance by the responsible professional and the patient or surrogate that the only way to achieve symptom relief is likely to involve sedating the patient until the patient is comfortable. In some cases, this may require sedation to unconsciousness.

A range of medications is used in palliative sedation. The amount of medication needed to provide symptom relief will vary according to the needs of the individual patient. Levels of sedation needed for symptom relief will range from light, to moderate, to sedation to unconsciousness, also according to the needs of the individual patient.

Palliative sedation requires the patient's or surrogate's informed consent. The goals of sedation, the plan for achieving these goals, and how symptom relief will be monitored clinically should be made clear to the patient with decision-making capacity (as well as to the patient without decision-making capacity when that is feasible), to the surrogate (if any), to loved ones, and to all staff involved in the care of this patient.

Palliative sedation also requires round-the-clock clinical vigilance to ensure continuous relief of symptoms without breakthrough pain or discomfort and may require rapid adjustments of medication. A dedicated palliative care unit or a clinical setting with close patient monitoring and palliative care expertise can provide the needed vigilance. Some organizations may be capable of administering palliative sedation outside of these settings.

Palliative sedation to relieve suffering in a patient who is close to death diminishes the consciousness of a patient who has no potential for recovery. There is general agreement among ethicists and palliative medicine specialists that palliative sedation, including sedation to unconsciousness, is justified when:

- a patient is expected to die as the result of the disease process irrespective of palliative sedation;
- the patient is experiencing pain or other symptoms that are intolerable to the patient;
- the pain or symptoms cannot be effectively managed using other palliative treatments;

- the goal of palliative sedation is the relief of the intolerable and refractory symptom(s), not to cause death, even though an unintended side effect of palliative sedation may be to hasten death in some cases;
- the patient or surrogate makes an informed choice to relieve symptoms using palliative sedation;
- a palliative medicine specialist or another clinician with expertise in the pharmacological treatment of pain and symptoms is responsible for introducing palliative sedation and for directing the care of the sedated patient until the patient's death; and
- the aim of the palliative sedation procedure is to titrate the dose of the sedating medication(s) until the symptom(s) are relieved.

### Relationship to withholding and withdrawing life-sustaining treatment—specifically, artificial (medically provided) nutrition and hydration

A decision to use palliative sedation to relieve intolerable symptoms is not by itself a decision to forgo life-sustaining treatment. However, a decision to institute palliative sedation may be part of a larger decision or set of decisions to forgo life-sustaining treatment, including ANH, to maintain comfort during the dying process. When a patient or surrogate has decided to forgo life-sustaining treatment, palliative sedation may sometimes be necessary to relieve symptoms and maintain comfort.

Conversely, once a patient or surrogate makes a decision to use palliative sedation to relieve intolerable symptoms, any decisions about starting or continuing life-sustaining interventions should be made in light of the patient's (or surrogate's) decision to use palliative sedation to relieve these symptoms. For example, starting or continuing ANH in such circumstances would usually only prolong the sedated state in a patient close to death and might well inflict burdens on the patient. In some dying patients hydration increases secretions, which may become difficult to manage. As a result, ANH is generally not part of the care plan for a dying patient who is undergoing palliative sedation, as the benefits fail to outweigh burdens.

### Education and policy supporting good practice in the use of palliative sedation

Many dying patients become less aware and even unconscious as their organs fail. Some treatments offered to seriously ill patients can also produce sedation as a side effect. By comparison, palliative sedation is a relatively rare form of medical treatment at the end of life. For palliative care and hospice clinicians, the availability of palliative sedation for intractable pain and symptoms is considered a necessary component of palliative care. Clinicians who work in settings where there is limited expertise in or experience with palliative medicine are likely to be much less familiar with this intervention.

As any physician or nurse who cares for patients who are forgoing life-sustaining treatment or nearing death may be called on to treat a patient who is experiencing refractory and intolerable pain or symptoms, these clinicians should have opportunities to learn about palliative sedation in the context of palliative care and in the broader context of good care at the end of life. These learning opportunities should include collaboration with specialists in palliative care, opportunities for training in palliative care, and opportunities to discuss the ethical dimensions of palliative sedation and current debates. To guide sound practice, institutional guidelines for palliative sedation should be in place. Creating these guidelines will call for collaboration among clinicians, experts in palliative care, and the ethics committee or others with ethics expertise. The Bibliography for this subsection includes a selection of practice recommendations and other recent literature for institutions to use in developing policy.

### Palliative sedation: Continuing debates

Education supporting good practice in the use of palliative sedation to relieve intractable pain or other physiological symptoms in a dying patient should also address continuing clinical and ethical debates in the United States and internationally about the conditions that may justify its use. Addressing these debates with clinicians helps clarify information and prevent misunderstandings, supports clear communication with patients and surrogates, and promotes ethical reflection.

One debate concerns the use of palliative sedation to relieve "existential suffering" in a dying patient. As discussed in Part Three, Section 3D ("Existential Suffering as a Factor in Treatment Decision-Making"), this term usually refers to suffering that is not relieved by the treatment of physiological symptoms or that occurs in the absence of such symptoms. The lack of a consensus definition of "existential suffering" presents a challenge for clinicians who seek to relieve the suffering of a dying patient who does not have refractory physiological symptoms. Some commentators argue that palliative sedation would relieve the patient's existential suffering by reducing the patient's awareness of his or her suffering. Other commentators argue that palliative sedation would greatly reduce the patient's remaining potential for meaningful social interaction with loved ones and other caregivers and that such social support may itself help relieve existential suffering for some patients. There is, as yet, no consensus among ethicists and palliative care specialists concerning the use of palliative sedation in response to existential suffering.

Opportunities for ethical reflection on this debate should include careful attention to current definitions of and clinical responses to existential suffering within the interdisciplinary palliative care literature. The literature specifically on palliative sedation is another resource, as it addresses clinical and ethical perspectives on this topic. The Bibliography for this section and for Part Three, Section 3, includes selections from these literatures.

Another debate concerns the acceptability of palliative sedation even if it risks hastening death in some patients. As discussed in these *Guidelines*, the available evidence suggests that it is actually rare that medication properly administered with the intent to relieve pain or symptoms will hasten a patient's death. (See Introduction, "Legal and Ethical Consensus.") In palliative sedation near the end of life, medication is titrated to the level required for comfort and is closely monitored. The expectation that the patient will die from an underlying disease process shortly after the introduction of palliative sedation does not mean that palliative sedation itself will hasten the patient's death. Even if there is a foreseeable risk that the use of sedation with the intent to relieve intolerable pain or symptoms will hasten death, it is ethically acceptable to properly administer the medication, as long as the intent is to relieve pain or symptoms (and not to end life) and the patient or surrogate has consented to the risks.

Opportunities for ethical reflection on this debate should include careful attention to the rule of double effect and its requirement that actions (such as precise titration and monitoring to ensure symptom relief) be consistent with the intent to relieve pain and symptoms, rather than an intent to use palliative sedation to end life. (On the rule of double effect, see Introduction, "Legal and Ethical Consensus.") The palliative care literature on the medical management of pain and symptoms near the end of life frequently addresses clinical and ethical perspectives and available empirical research on this topic. The Bibliography for this subsection, and for the Introduction, offers selections from this literature and scholarly commentary on the rule of double effect.

Opportunities for ethical reflection should also include careful attention to how palliative sedation for symptom relief in a patient who is near death differs from physician-assisted suicide or euthanasia, including in intent and clinical practice. The Bibliography for the Introduction includes a selection of recent literature on PAS and euthanasia that may further support education about palliative sedation in relation to these continuing ethical and social questions.

# Institutional Discussion Guide on Resource Allocation and the Cost of Care

## Introduction

Cost is an ethical issue in health care. The ethical goal of treating all patients equitably requires health care institutions to grapple with the moral as well as the fiscal dimensions of resource allocation and health care cost. Professionals need opportunities to discuss these difficult issues in an open and factually well-informed way, to prevent "bedside rationing" and other *ad hoc* resource allocation practices that are not transparent and that may be driven by priorities other than the provision of good care. They also need opportunities to discuss the economic impact of treatment decisions on patients and loved ones.

The relationship between financial considerations and decision-making about life-sustaining treatment and end-of-life care is too complex to lend itself to comprehensive ethics guidelines appropriate for all care settings. However, reflection on issues integral to ethical practice can aid in the development of policy that is ethically sound from a procedural standpoint. This section aims to help clinicians, administrators, trustees, and others involved in health care delivery and governance to discuss these issues in a structured and productive way. Developing an institutional practice of talking about the ethical dimensions of the cost of care aids in the development of policy to support the equitable allocation of limited resources. It also helps professionals with one of their most challenging problems: how to talk with patients and loved ones about treatment burdens that are economic.

This section offers six discussion strategies appropriate for senior leadership, medical directors, nursing directors, clinicians, staff, and ethics committees in hospitals, nursing homes, hospice programs, and home care agencies. These strategies are not examples of model policies. Rather, they offer suggestions for promoting well-informed discussion and consensus-building processes in preparation for developing policy appropriate for an individual institution's needs. Some of these strategies may also help an institution to air difficult resource allocation problems affecting its patient population.

These are challenging discussions for any institution. Professionals responsible for delivering care to patients who face decisions about life-sustaining treatment or are nearing the end of life should participate in these policy-making discussions to contribute their perspectives, raise questions that may not occur to nonclinicians, and enrich their own ethical and professional reflection on the work they do. Striving to achieve the ethical goal of equity requires professionals to protect seriously ill and dying patients from being denied access to resources based solely on a perception that a person who is ill or near the end of life has less social worth than another member of society. However, the interests of patients are not served solely through the quantity of treatment they receive. Patients have an interest in making sure that treatment accords with their preferences and meets the goals of their care. When patients or their surrogates refuse life-sustaining treatment, as addressed throughout these *Guidelines*, that refusal should be honored.

Controlling health care costs, setting priorities among medical treatments and services when not all services can be offered to all patients, and making resource allocation decisions at the institutional level present significant ethical and practical challenges. They will become even more important as life-sustaining treatment options multiply and the American population ages.

## A. Developing a Practice of Discussing Resource Allocation and the Cost of Care: Six Strategies

**Discussion strategy 1**

Provide an appropriate forum for discussing resource allocation.

Health care institutions should offer professionals and staff a constructive way to express their concerns about resource allocation, including practices that they observe and perceive to be unfair.[60] Institutions should aim to ensure that policy development is informed by insights from clinicians and paraprofessionals with direct responsibility for patient care. When an institution's resource allocation policies are handed down from senior executives without opportunities for discussion or appear to have been developed without clinician insights, these policies may produce *ad hoc* responses, such as "working the system" on behalf of some patients but not others. Policies that are not clearly stated and available to all may also become a source of moral distress for individual professionals and of continuing tension within teams and on units.

A well-functioning ethics committee, as described in Part Two, Section 6A ("Guidelines on Ethics Services in Institutions Providing Care for Patients Facing Decisions about Life-Sustaining Treatment or Approaching the End of Life") can provide this forum by regularly putting resource allocation on its discussion agenda, helping to develop institutional policy, and addressing cases that have triggered concerns over the fair distribution of resources. Discussion participants should be provided with accurate institutional data on costs. Staff members with special knowledge of legal and regulatory issues that may be relevant to resource allocation in a particular care setting can contribute to the analysis of these data and should be included in these discussions.

**Discussion strategy 2**

Describe the different levels at which health care resource allocation takes place. Support ethical reflection appropriate to each level, while clarifying which levels can be addressed by decisions within an institution.

In discussions of resource allocation, it is important to distinguish different decision-making and policy-making levels. Discussion facilitators can support participants by describing the following levels and identifying the level(s) relevant to their discussion:

### Large-scale, system-level resource allocation

Medicare and Medicaid financing, reimbursement rate setting, and health care reform legislation are examples of these large-scale issues. These resource allocation decisions are made at the federal and state levels and may have a powerful impact on life-sustaining treatment options as well as the delivery of end-of-life care, which is often financed heavily by Medicare. Discussing this level can provide important context for institutional decisions and policy.

### Institutional resource allocation: Investment decisions

Health care institutions make resource allocation decisions whenever they determine which service areas to invest in, maintain, or discontinue. As with large-scale resource allocation, these institutional decisions are values-based as well as economic, as an institution may demonstrate which services it values through its willingness or unwillingness to commit financial resources to a particular service. These decisions affect the care of patients who face decisions about life-sustaining treatment or are nearing the end of life when they involve institutional investment in services such as palliative care, which may not be fully reimbursable or may require upfront institutional investment in personnel and facilities. Another relevant category of institutional decisions is whether to continue or discontinue a service benefiting patients with life-threatening conditions. Typically these resource allocation decisions are made at a high level of institutional management and governance but should be informed by clinical perspectives.

### Institutional resource allocation: Admissions criteria and utilization rules

Institutions may allocate resources or seek to cap costs through admissions criteria and utilization rules. Policies concerning hospice admissions criteria, eligibility for dialysis, and utilization of repeated transfusions of whole blood are among many examples of resource allocation policies that affect patients who face decisions about life-sustaining treatment or are nearing the end of life. These resource allocation policies directly affect clinical practice.

Ethical concerns or interpersonal disagreements may arise when resource allocation policies conflict with patient preferences or when the rules for permitting or barring access to a scarce resource include nonmedical as well as medical criteria. Clinicians may disagree with resource allocation rules or become suspicious of the reasoning behind them. In such cases, they may attempt to resolve these concerns through *ad hoc* remedies that fall short of fair and transparent processes. Rules can be effective ways to limit variation and strive for equity of access. However, it is easy for staff to become cynical about rules that do not appear to be in patients' interests or that appear to benefit or protect one set of patients at the expense of another. For these reasons, resource allocation rules should be a frequent topic of discussion in institutions, with reference to ethical practice as well as institutional priorities.

## Institutional resource allocation: Care planning and treatment decision-making processes

The processes described in Part Two of these *Guidelines* allocate resources, in that they aim to prevent the delivery of unwanted or ineffective treatments. By doing this, the care-planning and decision-making processes strive to direct resources to those patients who want them, in keeping with the goals of their care.

### Discussion strategy 3

Identify known problems, shared goals, and viable options.

Discussion facilitators should describe a known resource allocation problem clearly and review past institutional patterns of deliberation and decision-making with the goal of identifying any flawed processes that may have contributed to this problem. Discussion participants should be encouraged to offer their perspectives on how to improve flawed processes and their ideas concerning the resource allocation problem at hand. Facilitators may ask selected participants to study a problem and return with recommendations, but should avoid suggesting to the group (or reporting to leadership) that these participants will be held responsible for "solving" a complex institutional problem.

### Discussion strategy 4

Develop a working vocabulary of concepts and definitions relevant to resource allocation.

Confusion over the definition of terms can make it hard to evaluate institutional resource allocation decisions, both economically and ethically. "Efficiency" is one such term. Allocating limited resources equitably involves reevaluation of practices that are inefficient because they waste resources, thereby further reducing the resources available to all patients. However, clinicians, like workers in other complex systems, may associate "efficiency" with pressure to increase productivity or revenue streams, rather than with efforts to use resources wisely. In some institutions, "efficiency" may be perceived as a euphemism for prioritizing the volume of reimbursable services over the quality of these services or the interests of individual patients. For example, a physician may observe and even participate in an institutional practice of ordering repeated diagnostic testing for patients near the end of life. This physician may conclude that this practice fails to deliver clear benefit for patients and represents a wasteful use of personnel and facilities. Different professions have different vocabularies and different values, which may influence how they view resource allocation questions; the language of "efficiency" may be familiar to an administrator but less familiar to a clinician. Discussion facilitators should provide participants with consensus definitions of terms such as "efficiency," "effectiveness," "benefit," "quality," "safety," "equity," "access," "stewardship," "limits," and other terms that may be associated with resource allocation in a health care institution. They should note the sources of these definitions, as well as any competing definitions and underlying concerns and values. Discussion participants should be encouraged to identify additional terms (and also practices, such as the use of generic drugs) that they may associate with resource allocation.

**Discussion strategy 5**

Provide information and training for professionals concerning the economic implications of treatment plans for patients and loved ones.

Physicians and other health care professionals may not be fully aware of the concrete economic implications of their treatment recommendations. Research suggests they may also be uncertain how to discuss these issues with patients, surrogates, and loved ones involved in a patient's care.[61] Physicians should not bear sole responsibility for addressing economic issues and should be able to rely on social workers and on institutional services to provide patients, surrogates, and loved ones with detailed information concerning insurance, entitlements, and other means of covering health care costs. However, to aid informed decision-making, physicians should be prepared to talk about costs associated with treatment options and recommendations, including out-of-pocket costs for treatments, technologies, or care arrangements that are not fully reimbursable. Physicians may find it useful to partner with others in the institution when communicating with patients, surrogates, and loved ones about treatment costs. Social workers, in particular, may have the needed knowledge and relevant communication experience, as they often work with patients and loved ones to resolve care problems related to insurance coverage or lack of insurance. Failure to address and compare the foreseeable costs of different treatment options may suggest to patients and loved ones that it is wrong to consider cost when assessing the benefits and burdens of treatment options, or that high cost is associated with high value. A growing body of empirical research and policy analysis on the high cost of treatments of uncertain or marginal benefit—particularly in the treatment of advanced cancer—and on the economic consequences of particular diagnoses for patients and family caregivers calls on clinicians and the institutions in which they work to recognize an obligation to provide patients and loved ones with clear information about out-of-pocket costs.[62] Institutions should support these efforts by helping professionals learn the facts about costs and how to discuss costs. The Bibliography supporting this section includes a selection of literature that can support clinician education on the cost of care and on discussing costs with patients, surrogates, and loved ones.

**Discussion strategy 6**

Conduct a survey or interviews to identify the resource allocation and cost issues that are most troubling to patient care professionals and staff within the institution. Address these issues in ongoing discussions. Develop ethics education programs that respond to specific needs.

An anonymous survey or confidential interviews will help those responsible for facilitating institutional discussions on resource allocation and the cost of care to identify those issues that are most troubling to an institution's professionals and staff. A survey or interview may also reveal knowledge gaps or misperceptions among staff with respect to current clinical outcomes of interventions involving limited resources, high cost, or both. Collecting information from a range of specialties and professions, and from paraprofessionals such as nurses' aides, will enrich the facilitators' understanding of how these issues are perceived and will increase the involvement of stakeholders in the discussion and policy development process.

## B. Discussing Uncompensated Care for Patients Without Insurance

The problem of uncompensated care can create ethical dilemmas for professionals, as they may face economic pressure to alter their care of individual patients who lack health care insurance or the ability to pay out-of-pocket.[63] Health care reform efforts at the national and state levels should ameliorate but will not fully solve this problem.

Health care professionals may be uncertain about their responsibilities when caring for uninsured patients who have the potential to benefit from chemotherapy, dialysis, or other life-sustaining treatments, or whose care needs may be appropriate for a nursing home they cannot afford. As discussed in these *Guidelines*, professionals should present all medically relevant treatment options so patients and surrogates can make informed choices among them. Being prepared to discuss treatment options with patients, surrogates, and loved ones may require the professional (or another team member, such as a social worker) to obtain information about financial assistance programs and other options that may exist for covering the cost of care. In some cases, the responsible professional may need to advocate within the institution for a patient to receive that care.

Cases in which patients need and want care for which funding is uncertain or absent may trouble the conscience of the individual professional and contribute to moral distress. They may lead to tension within teams, or between clinicians and management, due to competing beliefs about the right thing to do, whether for an individual patient or for patient subpopulations. Such cases may result in isolated problem-solving efforts, such as "bending the rules" on behalf of an individual patient or searching for a physician or institution willing to treat this patient for free. Institutional discussion should recognize the good intentions behind "bending the rules" while clarifying that these efforts are problematic because they may introduce inequities.

Institutional discussion and consensus-building will not solve the problem of how best to use an institution's limited resources to address the health care needs of patients who currently lack insurance. However, an institution should carefully address how it handles such cases, including pressures placed on clinicians to deny needed and desired care. The institution should have a clear way for a responsible health professional to advocate for needed and desired care for a patient without penalty to the patient or professional.

The components of a productive discussion about uncompensated care are as follows:

### 1. Present accurate facts

Discussion participants should share a baseline of information about the magnitude of the uncompensated care problem in the community served by the institution and in the institution itself, and about the financial implications of providing different types of uncompensated care. This baseline should include:

- how the institution defines "uncompensated care," and whether this definition includes upfront institutional investment in financial assistance programs or other services for patients who cannot afford to pay for health care;
- the dollar amount of the institution's most recent annual expenditures for uncompensated care, what these funds were used for, and what percentage of the institution's budget this amount represents; and
- the availability of state-level emergency Medicaid or other public or private "safety net" funding to cover health care for uninsured patients under certain conditions, and the extent to which this funding offsets uncompensated care needs in a community. For example, the availability of safety net funds and an institution's investment in social workers able to secure some health care coverage for uninsured patients may mean that some of these patients are represented in the institution's Medicaid reimbursements, rather than in its uncompensated care expenditures.

If the discussion will focus on ethical concerns in providing specific life-sustaining treatments as uncompensated care, such as dialysis or chemotherapy, the factual information provided should be relevant to these situations. Describing the medical, financial, and social aspects of the problem through the presentation of a representative case may be helpful.

### 2. Encourage expression of all views

The discussion facilitator should encourage participants to describe their values and perspectives concerning the allocation of institutional resources to cover uncompensated care, as such descriptions can help participants understand how different stakeholders view the same problem. However, the facilitator should try to identify shared values and promote consensus concerning ethical practice or policy recommendations. One discussion participant may express the belief that "once a patient is in the door, we have an obligation to provide all necessary care." Another participant may express the belief that "uncompensated care is a luxury we can't afford." The facilitator has a responsibility to correct misrepresentations of fact and to point out irreconcilable positions while helping all participants to appreciate the complexity of the problem. Thoughtful discussion of the ethical issues at stake involves the recognition that health care institutions have certain legal and ethical obligations to patients who cannot afford treatment and that individual health care professionals also have obligations to inform patients of all medically relevant treatment options, collaborate on sound decision-making with patients and surrogates, practice in keeping with relevant standards of care, and advocate for needed and desired care when necessary. At the same time, no patient has an unlimited right to health-related goods that are also needed by others.

### 3. Recognize that uncompensated care is a multi-level problem
The discussion facilitator should help participants to recognize that uncompensated care is a multi-level problem:

- Ethical concerns about the care of uninsured patients arise in part because of federal and state policy, as well as private employer and insurer decisions that result in restrictions on patients' access to insurance coverage and what the insurance will cover. This level of resource allocation usually cannot be altered or made up for at the institutional level. Institutional discussion and consensus-building should identify the large-scale factors that are relevant to the discussion at hand and whether there is any potential for the institution, on its own or in collaboration with other organizations, to challenge a policy that contributes to the problem.
- At the institutional management and governance level where decisions about institutional investments are made, the institution's senior leaders should recognize that the obligation to provide uncompensated care is integral to the mission of a health care institution. This obligation applies to for-profit, not-for-profit, and public institutions, as service in the public interest is a legal and an ethical condition of corporate status and licensure. At the same time, the obligation has practical limits. Those responsible for setting institutional priorities and for day-to-day operations need to be granted sufficient flexibility to allocate funds to cover uncompensated care and to deliberate concerning how to respond to growing demands and emerging needs equitably. An institutional discussion and consensus-building process may help develop policy recommendations concerning institutional investment in uncompensated care.
- The level of institutional admissions criteria and utilization rules is where clinicians are most likely to experience ethical concerns over uncompensated care. Clinicians

may perceive some institutional admissions criteria and utilization rules as contrary to good practice. Creating mechanisms for clinicians to advocate for individual patients' care needs and to participate in policy review and reconsideration are both important. Clinicians' proposals for modifying existing criteria and rules or crafting new policies may prompt institution-wide discussion and consensus-building.

- Institutional care planning and treatment decision-making processes may also ameliorate some institutional burdens associated with uncompensated care by reducing the potential for the delivery of unwanted or ineffective treatments. However, providing potentially effective and desired life-sustaining treatments that are costly and may be medically appropriate for an indefinite period may raise serious institutional challenges. Institutions in which these concerns arise will need to address the ethical and economic issues that arise, including allocation implications for other patients.

The situation of undocumented immigrants in the United States who have end-stage renal disease (ESRD) and who could benefit from dialysis but are not eligible for the Medicare entitlement available to cover this diagnosis and treatment because of their immigration status may be troubling to professionals who become involved in the diagnosis and treatment of these patients.[64] Access to specialty treatment for cancer and other conditions beyond the primary care scope of services available in community health programs open to undocumented immigrants is another recognized problem. Institutions in communities that include undocumented immigrants and other residents who lack adequate health care coverage should be prepared to address this issue; to identify the most equitable and compassionate options, including those that may be attainable through policy reforms (some of which are described in the Bibliography supporting this subsection); and to help professionals grapple with clinical situations that seem unfair.

# Notes

PREFACE TO THE SECOND EDITION

1. Bruce Jennings, Gregory E. Kaebnick, and Thomas H. Murray, eds., "Improving End-of-Life Care: Why Has It Been So Difficult?" *Hastings Center Report Special Report* 35, no. 6 (2005): S2–60.

INTRODUCTION

2. A "family," as this term is used in these *Guidelines*, may include close friends, or an intimate partner whose relationship to the person may or may not be recognized by law, as well as individuals with a biological or legal relationship to the patient. These *Guidelines* also use the term "loved ones" to encompass this range of relationships.

3. Margaret Campbell, Kathryn S. Bizek, and Mary Thill, "Patient Responses During Rapid Terminal Weaning from Mechanical Ventilation: A Prospective Study," *Critical Care Medicine* 27, no. 1 (1999): 73–77; Katri Elina Clemens, Ines Quednau, and Eberhard Klaschik, "Is There a Higher Risk of Respiratory Depression in Opioid-Naïve Palliative Care Patients during Symptomatic Therapy of Dyspnea with Strong Opioids?" *Journal of Palliative Medicine* 11, no. 2 (2008): 204–16; Susan B. LeGrand, Elias A. Khawam, Declan Walsh, and Nilo I. Rivera, "Opioids, Respiratory Function, and Dyspnea," *American Journal of Hospice and Palliative Care* 20, no. 1 (2003): 57–61.

4. See Oregon Public Health Division, *Oregon's Death with Dignity Act 2011 Annual Report*, pp. 1–3, at 1, 2, http://public.health.oregon.gov/ProviderPartnerResources/EvaluationResearch/DeathwithDignityAct/Pages/index.aspx. The corresponding 2011 data from Washington include seventy reported deaths that occurred after the ingestion of lethal medication. See Washington State Department of Health, *Washington State Department of Health 2011 Death with Dignity Act Report: Executive Summary*, pp. 1–12, at 1, http://www.doh.wa.gov/portals/1/Documents/5300/DWDA2011.pdf.

5. Of the sixty-one out of seventy-one Oregon deaths reported in 2011 for which hospice information was available, fifty-nine (96.7 percent) involved individuals enrolled in hospice, and two (3.3 percent) involved individuals not enrolled in hospice. (The hospice enrollment status of the remaining ten individuals was unknown.) Historically, 89.7 percent of all reported Oregon deaths have involved individuals confirmed as enrolled in hospice. See *Oregon's Death with Dignity Act 2011 Annual Report*, Table 1, p. 1. The corresponding 2011 data from Washington include fifty-eight individuals (83 percent) enrolled in hospice and eleven individuals (16 percent) not enrolled, with one whose hospice status was unknown. See *Washington State Department of Health 2011 Death with Dignity Act Report*, Table 5, p. 9.

PART ONE, "FRAMEWORK AND CONTEXT"

6. As used in these *Guidelines*, the term "nursing home" refers to a skilled nursing facility (SNF), a type of long-term care facility for individuals who require skilled nursing care, are often elderly and frail, and may be near the end of life due to one or more progressive health conditions. Many of the citations in the Bibliography that concern the health care needs of this population also use the term "nursing home." Nursing homes that care for residents who are near the end of life may also be home to younger residents who are not near the end of life and whose health care needs involve relatively stable health conditions. Nursing homes also provide subacute care to recently discharged hospital patients who may eventually return home.

7. According to the Centers for Disease Control and Prevention (CDC), the number of reported deaths in the United States in 2011 was 2,513,171. See Donna L. Hoyert and Jiaquan Xu, "Deaths: Preliminary Data for 2011," *National Vital Statistics Reports* 61, no. 6 (2012): 1–64, at 27, http://www.cdc.gov/nchs/deaths.htm. Accessed November 20, 2012.

8. According to 2001 data compiled by the CDC's National Center for Health Statistics and analyzed by researchers at the Brown University Center for Gerontology and Health Care Research, 49.5 percent of all U.S. deaths due to chronic illness occurred in a hospital, with significant variation among states. See *Facts on Dying: Policy Relevant Data on Care at the End of Life*, "USA and State Statistics: 2001 Data," at http://www.chcr.brown.edu/dying/2001data.htm; see also Andrea Gruneir, Vincent Mor, Sherry Weitzen, et al., "Where People Die: A Multilevel Approach to Understanding Influences on Site of Death in America," *Medical Care Research and Review* 64, no. 4 (2007): 351–78, at 361.

9. The 2004 National Nursing Home Survey estimated that one in five deaths in the United States occurred in a nursing home. See Anita Bercovitz, Frederic H. Decker, Adrienne Jones, and Robin E. Remsburg, "End-of-Life Care in Nursing Homes: 2004 National Nursing Home Survey," *National Health Statistics Reports* 9 (2008): 1–24, at 1, http://www.cdc.gov/nchs/data/nhsr/nhsr009.pdf. Accessed November 20, 2012.

10. In 2011, approximately 44.6 percent of deaths in the United States included hospice services. See National Hospice and Palliative Care Organization, "Fact and Figures: Hospice Care in America," 2012, pp. 1–18, at 4, http://www.nhpco.org/i4a/pages/index.cfm?pageid=5994. Accessed November 20, 2012.

11. According to the CDC, the ten leading causes of death in the United States in 2011 were, in order: diseases of heart (heart disease); malignant neoplasms (cancer); chronic lower respiratory diseases; cerebrovascular diseases (stroke); accidents (unintentional injuries); Alzheimer's disease; diabetes mellitus (diabetes); influenza and pneumonia; nephritis, nephrotic syndrome and nephrosis (kidney disease); and intentional self-harm (suicide). See Hoyert and Xu, "Deaths: Preliminary Data for 2011," at 28.

12. Carol E. Sieger, Jason F. Arnold, and Judith C. Ahronheim, "Refusing Artificial Nutrition and Hydration: Does Statutory Law Send the Wrong Message?" *Journal of the American Geriatrics Society* 50, no. 3 (2002): 544–50.

13. Susan E. Hickman, Charles P. Sabatino, Alvin H. Moss, and Jessica Wehrle Nester, "The POLST (Physician Orders for Life-Sustaining Treatment) Paradigm to Improve End-of-Life Care: Potential State Legal Barriers to Implementation," *Journal of Law, Medicine & Ethics* 36, no.1 (2008): 119–40.

## PART TWO, "GUIDELINES ON CARE PLANNING AND DECISION-MAKING"

### Section 1: "Guidelines for Advance Care Planning and Advance Directives: Using Patient Preferences to Establish Goals of Care and Develop the Care Plan"

14. A "chaplain," as this term is used in these *Guidelines*, refers either to a professional who has completed academic and clinical requirements and been certified to work in a health care setting by a recognized credentialing organization (such as the Association of Professional Chaplains) or to a supervised resident chaplain in an accredited clinical pastoral education (CPE) program. Board-certified chaplains can be of any faith and are trained to work in multifaith and multicultural settings. They are frequently involved in the care of patients nearing the end of life and often serve on interdisciplinary palliative care teams.

15. See http://respectingchoices.org; accessed November 20, 2012.

16. See http://www.epec.net and http://www.aacn.nche.edu/elnec; accessed November 20, 2012.

17. See http://www.alz.org; accessed November 20, 2012.

### Section 2: "Guidelines for the Decision-Making Process"

18. This process is described in Veterans Health Administration, VHA Handbook 1004.01, *Informed Consent for Clinical Treatments and Procedures,* paragraph 14c (1a–3d), effective August 17, 2009. This process is supported by VHA Handbook 1004.2 and VHA Handbook 1004.3, which include the VHA's guidelines for the implementation of a decision to withhold or withdraw life-sustaining treatment. These Handbooks are available at http://www.va.gov/vhapublications/; accessed November 20, 2012.

### Section 3: "Guidelines Concerning Neonates, Infants, Children, and Adolescents"

19. The adjective "pediatric" refers in these *Guidelines* to health care professionals and settings that serve minors facing decisions about life-sustaining treatment or care near the end of life. This usage is consistent with the American Academy of Pediatrics (AAP) and is not limited to children as distinct from adolescents. Both

children and adolescents may receive care from pediatric specialists (for example, pediatric cardiologists or pediatric oncologists) in pediatric settings.

20. The total number of reported deaths of infants (under the age of one year) that occurred in 2011 was 23,910, including 15,954 neonatal deaths (under twenty-eight days) and 7,956 postnatal deaths (twenty-eight days through eleven months). The total number of reported deaths of children and adolescents ages one through fourteen years that occurred in 2011 was 9,613, including 4,236 deaths from ages one to four years and 5,377 deaths from ages five to fourteen years. The CDC's preliminary report on deaths occurring in 2011 includes deaths of adolescents ages fifteen and older in the total deaths (29,624) occurring from ages fifteen through twenty-four years; in 2009, the most recent year for which adolescent deaths are broken out from adult deaths, there were 11,520 reported deaths of adolescents from ages fifteen to nineteen years. See Hoyert and Xu, "Deaths: Preliminary Data for 2011," at 31, 44, and Kenneth D. Kochanek, Jiaquan Xu, Sherry L. Murphy, Arialdi Miniño, and Hsiang-Ching Kung, "Deaths: Final Data for 2009," *National Vital Statistics Reports* 60, no. 3 (2011), 1–117, at 23 (Table 3), http://www.cdc.gov/nchs/data/nvsr/nvsr60/nvsr60_03.pdf. Accessed November 20, 2012.

21. See 45 C.F.R. part 46.408 in Cited Legal Authorities.

22. Current professional guidance from the American Academy of Pediatrics (AAP) defines the threshold of viability as twenty-two to twenty-five weeks. This is consistent with international definitions. See Hugh MacDonald and the Committee on Fetus and Newborn, "Perinatal Care at the Threshold of Viability," *Pediatrics* 110, no. 5 (2002): 1024–27, at 1024; and Maria Serenella Pignotti and Gianpaolo Donzelli, "Perinatal Care at the Threshold of Viability: An International Comparison of Practical Guidelines for the Treatment of Extremely Preterm Births," *Pediatrics* 121, no. 1 (2008): e193–98, at e193, http://pediatrics.aappublications.org/content/121/1/e193.full. Accessed November 20, 2012.

23. Jon E. Tyson, Nehal A. Parikh, John Langer, et al., "Intensive Care for Extreme Prematurity—Moving beyond Gestational Age," *New England Journal of Medicine* 358, no. 16 (2008): 1672–81, at 1678 (Tables A and B).

### Section 4: "Guidelines for Care Transitions"

24. See Bercovitz, Decker, Jones, and Remsburg, "End-of-Life Care in Nursing Homes: 2004 National Nursing Home Survey," at 1.

25. Ladislav Volicer, "End-of-Life Care for People with Dementia in Residential Care Settings," Alzheimer's Association, 2005, pp. 1–35, at 6, http://www.alz.org/national/documents/endoflifelitreview.pdf. Accessed November 20, 2012.

26. The 2004 National Nursing Home Survey reported that the average length of time since admission for all current residents was 835 days and that the median length of stay was 463 days. These figures may include short-term residents who are undergoing rehabilitation and residents who need custodial care in addition to residents who may be near the end of life. See Adrienne L. Jones, Lisa L. Dwyer, Anita R. Bercovitz, and Genevieve W. Strahan, "The National Nursing Home Survey: 2004 Overview," *National Center for Health Statistics Vital and Health Statistics* 13, no. 167 (2009): 1–155, at 4, http://www.cdc.gov/nchs/data/series/sr_13/sr13_167.pdf. Accessed November 20, 2012.

27. Diane E. Hoffman and Anita J. Tarzian. "Dying in America—an Examination of Policies That Deter Adequate End-of-life Care in Nursing Homes," *Journal of Law, Medicine & Ethics* 33, no. 2 (2005): 294–309.

28. Joan M. Teno, Susan L. Mitchell, Jonathan Skinner, et al., "Churning: The Association Between Health Care Transitions and Feeding Tube Insertion for Nursing Home Residents with Advanced Cognitive Impairment," *Journal of Palliative Medicine* 12, no. 4 (2009): 359–62; Vincent Mor, Orna Intrator, Zhanlian Feng, and David C. Grabowski, "The Revolving Door of Rehospitalization from Skilled Nursing Facilities," *Health Affairs* 29, no. 1 (2010): 57–64.

29. Gary E. Appelbaum, Joyce E. King, and Thomas E. Finucane, "The Outcome of CPR Initiated in Nursing Homes," *Journal of the American Geriatrics Society* 38, no. 3 (1990): 197–200. The overall survival rate for out-of-hospital cardiac arrest is 7.6 percent. See Comilla Sasson, Mary A.M. Rogers, Jason Dahl, and Arthur L. Kellerman, "Predictors of Survival from Out-of-Hospital Cardiac Arrest: A Systematic Review and Meta-Analysis," *Circulation: Cardiovascular Quality and Outcomes* 3 (2010): 63–81.

30. Appelbaum, King, and Finucane, "The Outcome of CPR Initiated in Nursing Homes," 197.

31. Some states and jurisdictions use terms other than "POLST" to refer to a program based on the POLST Paradigm. For a map of states and jurisdictions with POLST-type programs in place or in development with links to programs, see http://www.polst.org, "POLST Paradigm Programs"; accessed December 20, 2012.

32. The 2004 National Nursing Home Survey reported that 35.7 percent of current nursing home residents were admitted from an acute-care hospital, and 8.6 percent of residents were admitted from a hospital-based skilled nursing facility (44.3 percent total). An additional 23.2 percent of residents were admitted from other institutions, including other nursing homes or assisted living facilities. See Jones, Dwyer, Bercovitz, and Strahan, "The National Nursing Home Survey: 2004 Overview," at 22.

**Section 5: "Guidelines for the Determination of Death"**

33. President's Commission for the Study of Ethical Problems in Medicine and Biomedical and Behavioral Research, *Defining Death: Medical, Legal and Ethical Issues in the Determination of Death* (Washington, DC: Government Printing Office, 1981).

34. Eelco F.M. Wijdicks, Panayiotis N. Varelas, Gary S. Gronseth, and David M. Greer, "Evidence-Based Guideline Update: Determining Brain Death in Adults," *Neurology* 74, no. 23 (2010): 1911–18.

**Section 6: "Guidelines for Institutional Policy"**

35. This subsection is adapted with permission from Tia Powell and Jeffrey Blustein, "The Nature and Functioning of Ethics Committees," and Kenneth A. Berkowitz and Nancy Neveloff Dubler, "Approaches to Ethics Consultations," in Linda Farber Post, Jeffrey Blustein, and Nancy Neveloff Dubler, eds., *Handbook for Health Care Ethics Committees* (Baltimore, MD: Johns Hopkins University Press, 2007), 1–7, 139–53. Copyright holder's permission secured.

36. See American Society for Bioethics and Humanities, *Core Competencies for Health Care Ethics Consultation,* 2d ed. (Glenview, IL: American Society for Bioethics and Humanities, 2011).

37. Fitchett, George, *Assessing Spiritual Needs: A Guide for Caregivers* (Minneapolis, MN: Augsburg Fortress, 1993); Karen E. Steinhauser, Corinne I. Voils, Elizabeth C. Clipp, et al., "Are You at Peace? One Item to Probe Spiritual Concerns at the End of Life," *Archives of Internal Medicine* 166, no. 1 (2008): 101–5.

38. Nancy N. Dubler and Carol B. Liebman, *Bioethics Mediation: A Guide to Shaping Shared Solutions,* rev. ed. (Nashville, TN: Vanderbilt University Press/United Hospital Fund, 2011).

## PART THREE, "COMMUNICATION SUPPORTING DECISION-MAKING AND CARE"

**Section 1: "Communication with Patients, Surrogates, and Loved Ones"**

39. This subsection is adapted with permission from J. Randall Curtis, Donald L. Patrick, Sarah E. Shannon, et al., "The Family Conference as a Focus to Improve Communication about End-of-Life Care in the Intensive Care Unit: Opportunities for Improvement," *Critical Care Medicine* 29, no. 2, suppl. (2001): N26–33. Copyright holder's permission secured.

**Section 3: "Psychological Dimensions of Decision-Making about Life-Sustaining Treatment and Care Near the End of Life"**

40. Thomas J. Smith, Lindsay Dow, Enid Virago, et al., "Giving Honest Information to Patients with Advanced Cancer Maintains Hope," *Oncology* 24, no. 6 (2010): 521–25.

41. An earlier version of some material in this subsection appeared in Nancy Berlinger and Bruce Jennings, "Ethical Dilemmas and Spiritual Care Near the End of Life," in *Living with Grief: Spirituality and End-of-Life Care,* ed. Kenneth J. Doka and Amy S. Tucci (Washington, DC: Hospice Foundation of America, 2011), 49–62. Copyright holder's permission secured.

**Section 4: "Decision-Making Concerning Specific Treatments and Technologies"**

42. The authors wish to thank J. Randall Curtis, MD, MPH, of the project's working group, for providing unpublished material to aid in the initial drafting and subsequent revision of Sections 4A ("Forgoing Life-Sustaining Treatments: Ethical and Practical Considerations for Clinicians") and 4C ("Mechanical Ventilation"). Copyright holder's permission secured.

43. The authors wish to thank Joseph J. Fins, MD, FACP, of the project's working group, for providing unpublished material to aid in the initial drafting of this subsection. That material was subsequently published as Joseph J. Fins, "Brain Injury: The Vegetative and Minimally Conscious States," in *From Birth to Death and Bench to Clinic: The Hastings Center Bioethics Briefing Book for Journalists, Policymakers, and Campaigns* (Garrison, NY: The Hastings Center, 2008). Copyright holder's permission secured. The authors also wish to thank Kristi Kirschner, MD, of the project's working group, who participated in the further development of this subsection.

44. Bryan Jennet and Fred Plum, "Persistent Vegetative State after Brain Damage. A Syndrome in Search of a Name," *Lancet* 299, no. 7753 (1972): 734–37.

45. The Multi-Society Task Force on PVS, "Medical Aspects of the Persistent Vegetative State" (part 1), *NEJM* 330, no. 21 (1994): 1499–508.

46. Anna Estraneo, Pasquale Moretta, Vincenzo Loreto, et al., "Late Recovery after Traumatic, Anoxic, or Hemorrhagic Long-Lasting Vegetative State," *Neurology* 75, no. 3 (2010): 239–45.

47. Joseph T. Giacino, Stephen Ashwal, and Nancy Childs, "The Minimally Conscious State: Definition and Diagnostic Criteria," *Neurology* 58, no. 3 (2002): 349–53.

48. Some patients living with degenerative conditions use invasive mechanical ventilation noncontinuously, for example, by capping a tracheostomy when not in use. A range of other ventilation technologies may be used in chronic-care settings.

49. In some health care institutions, the DNR order is called a "do-not-attempt-resuscitation (DNAR) order" or an "allow-natural-death (AND) order." These variants may also be used in advance directive forms in some states. All refer to a medical order documenting the refusal of CPR specifically.

50. American Society of Anesthesiologists, "Ethical Guidelines for the Anesthesia Care of Patients with Do-Not-Resuscitate Orders or Other Directives that Limit Treatment," (approved 2001, affirmed 2008). Available at http://www.asahq.org. Accessed November 20, 2012.

51. Renal Physician Association, *Shared Decision-Making in the Appropriate Initiation and Withdrawal from Dialysis Clinical Practice Guidelines*, 2d ed. (Rockville, MD: Renal Physician Association, 2010).

52. Lewis M. Cohen, Michael J. Germain, and David M. Poppel, "Practical Considerations in Dialysis Withdrawal: 'To Have That Option Is a Blessing,'" *JAMA* 289, no. 16 (2003): 2113–19.

53. For a review of relevant research concerning the use of ANH in the contexts of ALS, cancer, and advanced dementia, see Linda Ganzini, "Artificial Nutrition and Hydration at the End of Life: Ethics and Evidence," *Palliative and Supportive Care* 4 (2006): 135–43.

54. Thomas E. Finucane, Colleen Christmas, and Kathy Travis, "Tube Feeding in Patients with Advanced Dementia: A Review of the Evidence," *JAMA* 282, no. 14 (1999): 1365–70. See also Jane Tilly, Peter Reed, Elizabeth Gould, and Abel Fok, *Dementia Care Practice: Recommendations for Assisted Living Residences and Nursing Homes, Phase 3: End of Life Care* (Chicago, IL: The Alzheimer's Association, 2007).

55. An earlier version of this material appeared in Nancy Berlinger and Bruce Jennings, "Ethical Dilemmas in the Treatment of Cancer," in *Living with Grief: Cancer and End-of-Life Care*, ed. Kenneth J. Doka and Amy S. Tucci (Washington, DC: Hospice Foundation of America, 2010), 83–96. Copyright holder's permission secured.

56. Jennifer S. Temel, Joseph A. Greer, Alona Muzikansky, et al., "Early Palliative Care for Patients with Metastatic Non-Small-Cell Lung Cancer," *NEJM* 368, no. 8 (2010): 733–42.

57. Robin Matsuyama, Sashidhar Reddy, and Thomas J. Smith, "Why Do Patients Choose Chemotherapy Near the End of Life? A Review of the Perspective of Those Facing Death from Cancer," *Journal of Clinical Oncology* 24, no. 21 (2006): 3490–96.

58. Stephen R. Connor, Bruce Pyenson, Kathryn Fitch, et al., "Comparing Hospice and Nonhospice Patient Survival among Patients Who Die within a Three-Year Window," *Journal of Pain and Symptom Management* 33, no. 3 (2007): 238–46. See also Temel, Greer, Muzikansky, et al. "Early Palliative Care for Patients with Metastatic Non-Small-Cell Lung Cancer."

59. The authors wish to thank Daniel Sulmasy, MD, PhD, FACP, and Nessa Coyle, ANP-BC of the project's working group, for providing unpublished material to aid in the initial drafting and subsequent revisions of this subsection. Copyright holders' permission secured.

**Section 5: "Institutional Discussion Guide on Resource Allocation and the Cost of Care"**
60. An earlier version of the material in this subsection appeared in Bruce Jennings and Mary Beth Morrissey, "Health Care Costs in End-of-Life and Palliative Care: The Quest for Ethical Reform," *Journal of Social Work in End-of-Life & Palliative Care* 7, no. 4 (2011): 300–17. Copyright holder's permission secured.

61. Peter J. Neumann, Jennifer A. Palmer, Eric Nadler, et al., "Cancer Therapy Costs Influence Treatment: A National Survey of Oncologists," *Health Affairs* 29, no. 1 (2010): 196–202.

62. Tito Fojo and Christine Grady, "How Much Is Life Worth: Cetuximab, Non-Small Cell Lung Cancer, and the $440 Billion Question," *Journal of the National Cancer Institute* 101, no. 15 (2009): 1044–48; Bruce E. Hillner and Thomas J. Smith, "Efficacy Does Not Necessarily Translate to Cost Effectiveness: A Case Study

in the Challenges Associated with 21st-Century Cancer Drug Pricing," *Journal of Clinical Oncology* 27, no. 13 (2009): 2111–13.

63. Council on Ethical and Judicial Affairs, American Medical Association, "Ethical Issues in Health Care Systems Reform: The Provision of Adequate Health Care," *JAMA* 272, no. 13 (1994): 1056–62.

64. Laura Hurley, Allison Kempe, Lori A. Crane, et al., "Care of Undocumented Individuals with ESRD: A National Survey of U.S. Nephrologists." *American Journal of Kidney Diseases* 53, no. 6 (2009): 940–49.

# Glossary

This Glossary includes brief definitions of terms used frequently throughout these *Guidelines* due to their broad relevance to treatment decision-making and care near the end of life. It also includes selected terms that are relevant in different end-of-life care settings.

Definitions and contextual discussions of many specialized terms can be found in Part Three, Section 4 ("Decision-Making Concerning Specific Treatments and Technologies"), and elsewhere in the text. Consult the Table of Contents and the Index to locate these definitions.

**Advance care planning** is a process for eliciting a patient's values and preferences concerning current or future medical treatment, using these preferences to establish the patient's goals of care, and developing and documenting a care plan that reflects patient preferences and can be modified so it remains consistent with changes in goals. Advance care planning may include the completion of proxy directives and/or treatment directives to guide care in the event that the patient loses decision-making capacity in the future. Advance care planning may also include the completion of portable medical orders.

An **advance directive** is a document in which a person who has decision-making capacity gives directions about future medical care, or designates who should make medical decisions for the person if he or she loses decision-making capacity in the future, or both. There are two types of advance directives: proxy directives and treatment directives.

**Artificial nutrition and hydration (ANH)**, also known as medically provided nutrition and hydration, is a set of life-sustaining treatments that deliver nutrients and/or fluids by means other than the mouth. An ANH intervention is often colloquially referred to as a "feeding tube."

The **best interests standard**, as the term is used in these *Guidelines*, refers to the standard for treatment decision-making by a surrogate on behalf of a patient without decision-making capacity, when the patient expressed no known treatment preferences while the patient had decision-making capacity and the patient's preferences cannot be inferred by the surrogate from their knowledge of and experience with the patient. The best interests standard is also the standard for treatment decision-making on behalf of a patient who has never had decision-making capacity and whose values and preferences cannot reliably be inferred by a surrogate. In the care of adult patients, the best interests standard is sometimes explained as what a "reasonable person" would choose if in the patient's circumstances.

**Cardiopulmonary resuscitation (CPR)** is a set of interventions undertaken at the time of a cardiac or respiratory arrest to restore heartbeat and breathing.

A **chronic condition** is a disease or disability that is long-lasting or recurrent.

Clinical ethics refers in these *Guidelines* to the practices by which an institution identifies, analyzes, discusses, and resolves or manages ethical issues arising in patient care. These practices include processes for the conduct of ethics consultations and the work of ethics committees. Clinical ethics also encompasses education for health care professionals who face ethically challenging situations as well as the development and review of institutional policies and procedures specific to decisions about life-sustaining treatment and end-of-life care.

Comfort care refers in these *Guidelines* to the care plan for a patient near the end of life, often following a decision to forgo life-sustaining treatment, in order to relieve pain and symptoms and ensure the patient's comfort.

A "do not resuscitate" (DNR) order is an order signed by a health care professional directing that no CPR efforts are to be undertaken in the event of a cardiac or respiratory arrest. A patient with a DNR order may choose to receive other forms of life-sustaining treatment and medical care.

A durable power of attorney for health care is an individual's written designation of another person to make health care decisions on his or her behalf if and when the individual loses decision-making capacity, when that designation is authorized by a state's durable power of attorney statute. A durable power of attorney is a type of proxy appointment document. A surrogate appointed through a durable power of attorney may be known as a "proxy" or an "agent."

An emancipated minor is an adolescent who is recognized by state law as living without the supervision of a parent or guardian, and who has the right to make their own medical decisions.

An emergency is a sudden, acute medical crisis requiring immediate medical attention to treat a patient's injury or serious impairment or to avoid death.

Ethics, as the term is used in these *Guidelines*, refers to critical reasoning about morality (right and wrong) in human conduct, with reference to principles and other standards. These *Guidelines* use the terms "ethics" and "morality" interchangeably.

Euthanasia, as this term is used in these *Guidelines*, refers to the intentional killing of a patient by a physician, as through the physician's administration of a lethal dose of medication. Euthanasia is permitted in some countries and is illegal in the United States.

Hand feeding, or supported oral feeding, is a procedure in which a patient is fed by another person who puts food into the patient's mouth, as by spoon or syringe.

Health care personnel are all persons involved in providing health care for patients. They include both health care professionals and health care workers such as nurses' aides.

A health care professional is a physician, nurse-practitioner, nurse, physician assistant, or other professional who provides health care.

The health care team includes all health care personnel involved in treating and caring for a particular patient.

Hospice care is a team-oriented approach to medical care, pain and symptom management, and emotional and spiritual support tailored to the preferences and needs of a patient near the end of life. An adult becomes eligible for the Medicare Hospice Benefit once a physician certifies that the patient is terminally ill with a life expectancy of six months or less if the disease process follows its normal course and the patient forgoes further curative treatment aimed at the terminal disease process. Hospice care for children and adults eligible for Medicaid may be covered by Medicaid, and most private insurers also cover hospice care. Hospice care can be provided at home, in hospitals and nursing homes, and in other settings.

A life-sustaining treatment is any medical intervention administered to a patient with the goal of prolonging life and delaying death.

A life-threatening condition is a disease or injury that has a high likelihood of resulting in death if untreated, or if life-sustaining interventions are forgone or do not succeed.

For living will, see treatment directive.

A mature minor is an adolescent who is recognized by law as having the ability to make informed decisions about his or her own health care.

Medical refers in these *Guidelines* to the treatment of diseases or health conditions by health care professionals. It is not used here to refer to the concerns and practice of physicians exclusively.

Medical ethics refers in these *Guidelines* to ethics in the medical context, including the practice of health care professionals other than physicians.

Pain and symptom relief is the relief of suffering through the use of medication and other interventions to control pain and symptoms.

Palliative care refers in these *Guidelines* to pain and symptom relief and the care of the patient as a whole person and a social being during the experience of illness, including during medical treatment. It includes but is not limited to hospice care and comfort care near death.

Physician-assisted suicide (PAS), as this term is used in these *Guidelines*, refers to a practice currently authorized by statute in two states in the United States that permits terminally ill state residents under certain conditions to obtain from a physician a prescription for a lethal dose of medication for voluntary self-administration. PAS is sometimes referred to as "assisted suicide," "physician aid-in-dying," or "physician-assisted death."

Portable medical orders are documents that reflect the care plan agreed to by the patient or surrogate in the form of medical orders signed by a physician or other authorized health care professional, which can guide a patient's treatment and care across care settings. They are typically used for seriously ill patients facing foreseeable medical crises and care transitions. A set of portable medical orders produced through a Physician Orders for Life-Sustaining Treatment care planning process is often referred to as a POLST.

A progressive condition is a disease or disability that worsens over time. The outcome of a progressive condition that follows its normal course may be death.

A proxy directive is an individual's written designation of another person to make health care decisions on behalf of the designating individual in the event that he or she becomes incapable of making decisions.

The responsible health care professional is the health care professional with primary responsibility for directing a patient's medical treatment and care. Typically this is a physician. Sometimes it is a nurse-practitioner, nurse, physician assistant, or a physician-nurse team. The identity of the responsible health care professional may change during the course of a patient's treatment and care.

The substituted judgment standard, as the term is used in these *Guidelines*, refers to the standard for treatment decision-making by a surrogate on behalf of a patient without decision-making capacity, when the patient stated no explicit treatment preferences when the patient had decision-making capacity, but the patient's treatment preferences can be inferred by the surrogate from his or her knowledge of and experience with the patient.

A surrogate is an individual whose role is to make health care decisions for another person who lacks decision-making capacity. Individuals can use proxy appointment documents to state who should act as their surrogate if they lose decision-making capacity in the future. A surrogate appointed in this way may be known as a "proxy" or an "agent." Some states have laws for the identification of a default surrogate, such as a spouse or adult child, when the patient has not previously designated who should act as their surrogate. Some states also authorize surrogate decision-making committees to fulfill the surrogate role for some patients who lack individual surrogates (often called "unbefriended" patients). Health care institutions may also have surrogate decision-making processes for patients who lack individual surrogates. Note that establishing a surrogate for a patient who lacks one and who has lost decision-making capacity may call for legal consultation and require judicial intervention. A court-appointed surrogate is known as a "guardian" or a "conservator."

Terminally ill means having an incurable or irreversible condition that has a high probability of causing death within a relatively short time with or without treatment.

A treatment directive is a written statement by an individual stating what forms of medical treatment the individual wishes to receive or forgo under specified medical conditions (such as irreversible unconsciousness, severe and irreversible dementia, or terminal illness) if the individual loses decision-making capacity. A "living will" is one type of treatment directive. Note that an individual's oral instructions are also recognized as valid instructions even if not documented in the form of a treatment directive.

# Cited Legal Authorities

For a comprehensive roster of cases relevant to the right to forgo medical treatment, and other resources useful to legal counsel and to policy-makers, see Alan Meisel and Kathy L. Cerminara, *The Right to Die: The Law of End-of-Life Decisionmaking*, 3d ed. (New York: Aspen Publishers, 2004), and annual cumulative supplements.

See also the Selected Bibliography.

## CASES

*Baxter v. Montana*, No. ADV-2007–787, 2008 WL 6627324 (Mont. Dist. 2008), *aff'd in part*, 2009 MT 449, 354 Mont. 234, 224 P.3d 1211 (2009).

*Cruzan v. Dir., Mo. Dept. of Health*, 497 U.S. 261 (1990).

*In re Quinlan*, 70 N.J. 10, 355 A.2d 647, *cert. denied*, 429 U.S. 922 (1976).

*Nat'l Fed'n of Indep. Bus. v. Sebelius*, 132 S.Ct. 2566 (2012).

*Vacco v. Quill*, 521 U.S. 793 (1997).

*Washington v. Glucksberg*, 521 U.S. 702 (1997).

## STATUTES

### State statutes

Oregon Death with Dignity Act, OR. REV. STAT. §§ 127.800–.995 (2011).

Washington Death with Dignity Act, WASH. REV. CODE. §§ 70.245.010–.904 (2010).

### Federal statutes

Emergency Medical Treatment and Active Labor Act, 42 U.S.C.A. § 1395dd (West 2012).

Federal Nursing Home Reform Act, enacted as part of the Omnibus Budget Reconciliation Act of 1987, Pub. L. No. 100203, §§ 4201–4218, 101 Stat. 1330, 1330–160 to 1330–221 (2000) (codified at 42 U.S.C. §§ 1395i-3, 1396r (2006 & Supp. IV 2011)).

Omnibus Budget Reconciliation Act of 1990, Pub. L. 101–508, §§ 4206, 4751, 104 Stat. 1388, 1388–115, 1388–204 (1990) (known as the Patient Self-Determination Act).

Patient Protection and Affordable Care Act, Pub. L. No. 111–148, 124 Stat. 119 (2010) (codified as amended in scattered sections of 26 and 42 U.S.C.).

*Model statutes*

REV. UNIF. ANATOMICAL GIFT ACT (2006), 8A U.L.A. 46 (Supp. 2012).
UNIF. DETERMINATION OF DEATH ACT (1980), 12A U.L.A. 781 (2008).

## REGULATIONS

Conditions for Coverage of Suppliers of End-Stage Renal Disease Services, 42 C.F.R. §§ 405.2102–.2113 (2011).
Medicare and Medicaid Programs: Hospice Conditions of Participation, 42 C.F.R. pt. 418 (2011) (known as the
    Medicare Hospice Benefit).
Protection of Human Subjects, 45 C.F.R. pt. 46 (2011) (known as the Common Rule).

# Selected Bibliography

Empirical research on most of the topics discussed in these *Guidelines* is ongoing. We cite key studies below, offering health care professionals and other personnel opportunities to use recent studies to aid in ethical reflection, ethics education, and policy development, as well as to apply research findings to clinical practice and the organization of care. We also cite pronouncements by relevant professional societies and other membership organizations. Such organizations may consider ethics questions in the context of clinical practice guidelines and other consensus statements, and often incorporate some level of ethical analysis or guidance into these documents.

Understanding the ethical and practical complexity of end-of-life care is enriched by reading beyond one's own specialty or professional literature. This Bibliography lists a number of sources that we have found to be especially useful or thought-provoking in revising and updating these *Guidelines*, as well as some historically important documents. We do not attempt to list all of the documents available on the topics we address. Many of the sources for the Introduction and Part One also provide background for the decision-making guidelines and other topical sections and subsections that follow.

The websites listed below offer many additional citations for research studies and educational materials.

We use the following abbreviations in journal citations:

*JAMA: Journal of the American Medical Association*
*NEJM: New England Journal of Medicine*

## SELECTED WEBSITES ON TREATMENT DECISION-MAKING AND END-OF-LIFE CARE

Search terms in quotations are provided as finding aids and refer to the location of relevant material within multi-topic websites. Terms and locations are current as of June 11, 2012.

Agency for Healthcare Research and Quality (AHRQ): www.ahrq.gov

- "End of Life Care" subdirectory includes link to AHRQ-funded studies of advance care planning, with citations to empirical research

Alzheimer's Association: www.alz.org

- helpline (1–800–272–3900) is toll-free and staffed twenty-four hours a day, seven days a week, for patients, loved ones, and professionals
- helpline offers confidential care consultation by masters-level clinicians, and information on available services
- website includes information on advance care planning (including financial planning), written for the person with early-stage Alzheimer's disease
- "Professionals" area includes practice recommendations for end-of-life care in assisted living facilities and nursing homes
- "Facts and Figures" reports include annual data on Alzheimer's disease and other dementia in the United States and each state

American Bar Association (ABA): www.americanbar.org

- "Commission on Law and Aging" includes list of ABA publications on topics including "health care: decisionmaking"

Center to Advance Palliative Care (CAPC): www.capc.org

Dartmouth Atlas of Healthcare: www.dartmouthatlas.org

- key topics include "End-of-Life Care"
- website includes datasets for key topics

Education in Palliative and End-of-life Care (EPEC): www.epec.net

- EPEC for Veterans curriculum addresses relevance of combat history to care planning

End-of-Life Nursing Education Consortium (ELNEC): www.aacn.nche.edu/elnec

- ELNEC for Veterans curriculum addresses relevance of combat history to care planning

End of Life/Palliative Education Resource Center (EPERC): www.eperc.mcw.edu

*Handbook for Rural Health Care Ethics: A Practical Guide for Professionals*: http://geiselmed.dartmouth.edu/cfm/resources/ethics/

- website houses full text of the *Handbook*, which includes chapters on end-of-life decision-making and related topics, plus a selected bibliography

The Hastings Center: www.thehastingscenter.org

Hospice Foundation of America: www.hospicefoundation.org

- website includes downloadable versions of HFA's *Living with Grief* annual book series and other educational resources for professionals, paraprofessionals, and family caregivers

Initiative for Pediatric Palliative Care (IPPC): www.ippcweb.org

- website for interdisciplinary pediatric palliative care educational program offers twenty-five hours of peer-reviewed and field-tested instructional materials, including cases, slide sets, and films on DVD
- topics include improving communications with patients and families, relieving pain and symptoms, analyzing ethical challenges, and responding to suffering and bereavement

Lambda Legal: www.lambdalegal.org

- includes "Tools for Protecting Your Health Care Wishes," a publication offering detailed information on advance directives (including hospital visitation directives) for LGBT patients and their loved ones

*The Merck Manual Online*: www.merckmanuals.com/professional

- "Special Subjects" include the "Dying Patient," written by Joanne Lynn, MD, MA, MS

National Center for Ethics in Health Care: www.ethics.va.gov

- "Catalog of NCEHC Material" offers publications on many topics relevant to treatment decision-making and care near the end of life, including processes for ethics consultation and for surrogate decision-making for patients who lack decision-making capacity and also lack surrogates
- for VHA Handbooks: www.va.gov/vhapublications/

National Center for Health Statistics: www.cdc.gov/nchs

- "National Health Care Surveys" includes results of the National Nursing Home Survey, the National Hospice and Home Care Survey, and surveys of other care settings and professional and paraprofessional workforces involved in care near the end of life
- "National Health Care Surveys" also includes summaries of survey data on topics such as the prevalence of different types of advance directives among different long-term care populations
- "National Vital Statistics System" includes mortality data for the United States and for geographic areas within the United States

National Consensus Project for Quality Palliative Care: www.nationalconsensusproject.org

- website houses *Clinical Practice Guidelines for Quality Palliative Care*, 2d ed. (2009)

National Guideline Clearinghouse: http://guidelines.gov/

National Hospice and Palliative Care Organization: (NHPCO): www.nhpco.org

- "Hospice Statistics and Research" page includes links to annual "Facts and Figures" reports on hospice utilization in the United States
- "Caring Connections" portal includes link to state-specific advance directive forms

Respecting Choices: http://respectingchoices.org/

Physician Orders for Life-Sustaining Treatment Paradigm (POLST Paradigm): www.polst.org

Uniform Law Commission: www.uniformlaws.org

## INTRODUCTION

Burt, Robert A. *Death Is That Man Taking Names: Intersections of American Medicine, Law, and Culture*. Berkeley: University of California Press, 2002.

Cassell, Eric J. *The Nature of Suffering and the Goals of Medicine*. 2d ed. New York: Oxford University Press, 2004.

Cohen, Cynthia B., ed. *Casebook on the Termination of Life-Sustaining Treatment and the Care of the Dying*. Bloomington: Indiana University Press, 1988.

Field, Marilyn J., and Richard E. Behrman, eds. *When Children Die: Improving Palliative and End-of-Life Care for Children and Their Families*. Washington, DC: Institute of Medicine, National Academies Press, 2003.

Field, Marilyn J., and Christine K. Cassel, eds. *Approaching Death: Improving Care at the End of Life*. Washington, DC: Institute of Medicine, National Academies Press, 1998.

Jennings, Bruce, Gregory E. Kaebnick, and Thomas H. Murray, eds. "Improving End-of-Life Care: Why Has It Been So Difficult?" Hastings Center Report, Special Report 35, no. 6 (2005): S2–60.

Jennings, Bruce, True Ryndes, Carol D'Onofrio, and Mary Ann Baily. "Access to Hospice Care: Expanding Boundaries, Overcoming Barriers." Hastings Center Report, Special Report 33, no. 2 (2003): S1–60.

Lynn, Joanne. *Sick To Death and Not Going to Take It Anymore! Reforming Health Care for the Last Years of Life*. Berkeley: University of California Press, 2004.

Kaufman, Sharon. *…And a Time to Die: How American Hospitals Shape the End of Life*. New York: Scribner, 2005.

Moskowitz, Ellen H., and James Lindemann Nelson, eds. "Dying Well in the Hospital: The Lessons of SUPPORT." Hastings Center Report Special Supplement, 25, no. 6 (1995): S3–36.

Nuland, Sherwin B. *How We Die: Reflections on Life's Final Chapter*. New York: Knopf, 1994.

Staton, Jana, Roger Shuy, and Ira Byock. *A Few Months to Live: Different Paths to Life's End*. Washington, DC: Georgetown University Press, 2001.

SUPPORT Principal Investigators. "A Controlled Trial to Improve Care for Seriously Ill Hospitalized Patients: The Study to Understand Prognoses and Preferences for Outcomes and Risks of Treatments," JAMA 274, no. 20 (1995): 1591–98.

The Hastings Center. *Guidelines on the Termination of Life-Sustaining Treatment and the Care of the Dying*. Bloomington: Indiana University Press, 1987.

## LEGAL AND ETHICAL CONSENSUS/KEY DISTINCTIONS

### Right to refuse treatment

Meisel, Alan. "The Legal Consensus about Forgoing Life-Sustaining Treatment: Its Status and Prospects," Kennedy Institute of Ethics Journal 2, no. 4 (1993): 309–45.

Meisel, Alan, and Kathy L. Cerminara. *The Right to Die: The Law of End-of-Life Decisionmaking*. 3d ed. New York: Aspen Publishers, 2004, and annual cumulative supplements.

Meisel, Alan, Lois Snyder, and Timothy E. Quill. "Seven Legal Barriers to End-of-Life Care: Myths, Realities, and Grains of Truth." JAMA 284, no. 19 (2000): 2495–2501.

### Surrogate decision-making

Buchanan, Allen E., and Dan W. Brock. *Deciding for Others: The Ethics of Surrogate Decision Making*. New York: Cambridge University Press, 1990.

President's Commission for the Study of Ethical Problems in Medicine and Biomedical and Behavioral Research. *Making Health Care Decisions: A Report on the Ethical and Legal Implications of Informed Consent in the Patient-Practitioner Relationship*. Washington DC: U.S. Government Printing Office, 1982.

### Withholding and withdrawing life-sustaining treatment

American Medical Association Council on Ethical and Judicial Affairs, Opinion 2.20. "Withholding or Withdrawing Life-Sustaining Treatment." Chicago, IL: American Medical Association, 1994. Available at: www.ama-assn.org, "AMA Code of Medical Ethics."

President's Commission for the Study of Ethical Problems in Medicine and Biomedical and Behavioral Research. *Deciding to Forego Life-Sustaining Treatment: Ethical, Medical, and Legal Issues in Treatment Decisions*. Washington, DC: U.S. Government Printing Office, 1983.

Solomon, Mildred Z, Lydia O'Donnell, Bruce Jennings, Vivian Guilfoy, Susan M. Wolf, Kathleen Nolan, Rebecca Jackson, Dieter Koch-Weser, and Strachan Donnelley. "Decisions Near the End of Life: Health Care Professionals' Views on the Use of Life-Sustaining Medical Treatments." American Journal of Public Health 83, no. 1 (1993): 14–23.

### Ordinary and extraordinary/benefits and burdens
Meisel, Alan. "Legal Myths about Terminating Life Support." Archives of Internal Medicine 151, no. 8 (1991): 1497–1502.
Sulmasy, Daniel P. "Terri Schiavo and the Roman Catholic Tradition of Forgoing Extraordinary Means of Care." Journal of Law, Medicine & Ethics 33, no. 2 (2005): 359–62.

### Palliative care
Lynn, Joanne, Ekta Chaudhry, Lin Noyes Simon, Anne M. Wilkinson, and Janice Lynch Schuster. The Common Sense Guide to Improving Palliative Care. 2d ed. New York: Oxford University Press, 2007.
Meier, Diane E., Stephen L. Isaacs, and Robert Hughes, eds. Palliative Care: Transforming the Care of Serious Illness. San Francisco, CA: Robert Wood Johnson Foundation Health Policy Series/Jossey-Bass, 2010.
Temel, Jennifer S., Joseph A. Greer, Alona Muzikansky, Emily R. Gallagher, Sonal Admane, Vicki A. Jackson, Constance M. Dahlin, Craig D. Blinderman, Juliet Jacobsen, William F. Pirl, J. Andrew Billings, and Thomas J. Lynch. "Early Palliative Care for Patients with Metastatic Non-Small-Cell Lung Cancer." NEJM 368, no. 8 (2010): 733–42.

### Double effect
Campbell, Margaret, Kathryn S. Bizek, and Mary Thill. "Patient Responses during Rapid Terminal Weaning from Mechanical Ventilation: A Prospective Study." Critical Care Medicine 27, no. 1 (1999): 73–77.
Clemens, Katri Elina, Ines Quednau, and Eberhard Klaschik. "Is There a Higher Risk of Respiratory Depression in Opioid-Naive Palliative Care Patients during Symptomatic Therapy of Dyspnea with Strong Opioids?" Journal of Palliative Medicine 11, no. 2 (2008): 204–16.
LeGrand, Susan B., Elias A. Khawam, Declan Walsh, and Nilo I. Rivera. "Opioids, Respiratory Function, and Dyspnea." American Journal of Hospice and Palliative Care 20, no. 1 (2003): 57–61.
Sulmasy, Daniel P., and Edmund D. Pellegrino. "The Rule of Double Effect: Clearing Up the Double Talk." Archives of Internal Medicine 159, no. 6 (1999): 545–50.

### Physician-assisted suicide and euthanasia
Campbell, Courtney S., and Jessica C. Cox. "Hospice and Physician-Assisted Death: Collaboration, Compliance, and Complicity." Hastings Center Report 40, no. 5 (2010): 26–35.
Foley, Kathleen M., and Herbert Hendin, eds. The Case against Assisted Suicide: For the Right to End-of-Life Care. Baltimore, MD: Johns Hopkins University Press, 2002.
Quill, Timothy E., and Margaret P. Battin, eds. Physician-Assisted Dying: The Case for Palliative Care and Patient Choice. Baltimore, MD: Johns Hopkins University Press, 2004.
Robinson, John. "Baxter and the Return of Physician-Assisted Suicide." Hastings Center Report 40, no. 6 (2010): 15–17.
Tolle, Susan W., Virginia R. Tilden, Linda L. Drach, Erik K. Fromme, Nancy A. Perrin, and Katrina Hedberg. "Characteristics and Proportion of Dying Oregonians Who Personally Consider Physician-Assisted Suicide." Journal of Clinical Ethics 15, no. 2 (2004): 111–18.
Wolf, Susan M. "Assessing Physician Compliance with the Rules for Euthanasia and Assisted Suicide." Archives of Internal Medicine 165 (2005): 1677–79.
———. "Confronting Physician-Assisted Suicide and Euthanasia: My Father's Death." Hastings Center Report 38, no. 5 (2008): 23–26.
———. "Gender, Feminism, and Death: Physician-Assisted Suicide and Euthanasia." In: Feminism and Bioethics: Beyond Reproduction, ed. Susan M. Wolf. New York: Oxford University Press, 1996, pp. 282–317.
———. "Physician-Assisted Suicide." Clinics in Geriatric Medicine 21 (2005): 179–92.
———. "Pragmatism in the Face of Death: The Role of Facts in the Assisted Suicide Debate." Minnesota Law Review 82 (1998): 1063–2101.

PART ONE: FRAMEWORK AND CONTEXT

*Section 1: Ethics Goals, and Section 2: Ethics Education Competencies*

Browning, David, and Mildred Z. Solomon. "The Initiative for Pediatric Palliative Care: An Interdisciplinary Educational Approach for Health Care Professionals." Journal of Pediatric Nursing 20, no. 5 (2005): 326–34.

Carter, Brian S., Marcia Levetown, and Sarah E. Friebert, eds. *Palliative Care for Infants, Children, and Adolescents.* 2d ed. Baltimore: Johns Hopkins University Press, 2011.

Duke Institute on Care at the End of Life. *Key Topics on End-of-Life Care for African-Americans.* Durham, NC: Duke Institute on Care at the End of Life, 2006. Available at: http://divinity.duke.edu/initiatives-centers/iceol/resources/last-miles.

Ford, Paul J., and Denise M Dudzinski, eds. *Complex Ethics Consultations: Cases That Haunt Us.* New York: Cambridge University Press, 2008.

Lo, Bernard. *Resolving Ethical Dilemmas: A Guide for Clinicians.* 4th ed. Philadelphia, PA: Wolters Kluwer Health/Lippincott Williams and Wilkins, 2009.

Lynn, Joanne, Joan Harrold, and Janice Lynch Schuster. *Handbook for Mortals: Guidance for People Facing Serious Illness.* 2d ed. New York: Oxford University Press, 2011.

Nelson, William A., ed. *Handbook for Rural Health Care Ethics: A Practical Guide for Professionals.* Lebanon, NH: Dartmouth College Press/University Press of New England, 2009.

Post, Linda Farber, Jeffrey Blustein, and Nancy N. Dubler. *Handbook for Health Care Ethics Committees.* Baltimore, MD: Johns Hopkins University Press, 2007.

Snyder, Lois, and Timothy E. Quill, eds. *Physician's Guide to End-of-Life Care.* Philadelphia, PA: American College of Physicians, 2001.

Solomon, Mildred Z., David Browning, Deborah Dokken, Melanie Merriman, and Cynda Rushton. "Learning That Leads to Action: Impact and Characteristics of a Professional Education Approach to Improve the Care of Critically Ill Children and Their Families." Archives of Pediatric and Adolescent Medicine 164, no. 4 (2010): 315–22.

*Section 3: Organizational Systems*

Dixon-Woods, Mary, Charles L. Bosk, Emma Louise Aveling, Christine A. Goeschel, and Peter J. Provonost. "Explaining Michigan: Developing an Ex Post Theory of a Quality Improvement Program." Milbank Quarterly 89, no. 2 (2011): 167–205.

Farquhar, Cynthia M., Emma W. Kofa, and Jean R. Slutsky. "Clinicians' Attitudes to Clinical Practice Guidelines: A Systematic Review." Medical Journal of Australia 177, no. 9 (2002): 502–6.

Lynn, Joanne, Janice Lynch Schuster, Anne M. Wilkinson, and Lin Noyes Simon. *Improving Care for the End of Life: A Handbook for Health Care Managers and Clinicians.* 2d ed. New York: Oxford University Press, 2008.

Lynn, Joanne, Kevin Nolan, Andrea Kabcenell, David Weissman, Casey Milne, and Donald M. Berwick. "Reforming Care for Persons Near the End of Life: The Promise of Quality Improvement." Annals of Internal Medicine 137, no. 2 (2002): 117–22.

Solomon, Mildred Z., Anna Romer, Deborah Sellers, Bruce Jennings, and Steven Miles for The National Task Force on End-of-Life Care in Managed Care. "Meeting the Challenge: Twelve Recommendations for Improving End-of-Life Care in Managed Care." Newton, MA: Education Development Center, 1999. Available at: http://www.rwjf.org/reports/grr/036375s.htm.

*Section 4: Social, Economic, and Legal Contexts*

Brock, Dwight B., and Daniel J. Foley. "Demography and Epidemiology of Dying in the U.S. with Emphasis on Deaths of Older Persons." Hospice Journal 13, nos. 1–2 (1998): 49–60.

Flory, James, Young-Xu Yinong, Ipek Gurol, Norman Levinsky, Arlene Ash, and Ezekiel Emanuel. "Place of Death: U.S. Trends since 1980." Health Affairs 23, no. 3 (2004): 194–200.

Gillick, Muriel R. "How Medicare Shapes the Way We Die." Journal of Health & Biomedical Law 8 (2012): 27–55.

Goodman, David C., Amos R. Esty, Elliott S. Fisher, and Chiang-Hua Chang. *Trends and Variation in End-of-Life Care for Medicare Beneficiaries with Severe Chronic Illness.* Hanover, NH: The Dartmouth Institute for Health Policy and Clinical Practice, 2011.

Gruneir, Andrea, Vincent Mor, Sherry Weitzen, Rachel Truchil, Joan Teno, and Jason Roy. "Where People Die: A Multilevel Approach to Understanding Influences on Site of Death in America." Medical Care Research and Review 64, no. 4 (2007): 351–78.

Murray, Christopher J.L., Sandeep C. Kulkarni, Catherine Michaud, Niels Tomijima, Maria T. Bulzacchelli, Terrell J. Iandiorio, and Majid Ezzati. "Eight Americas: Investigating Mortality Disparities across Races, Counties, and Race-Counties in the United States." Public Library of Science Medicine 3, no. 9 (2006): e260. Available at: http://www.plosmedicine.org/article/info:doi/10.1371/journal.pmed.0030260.

Sieger, Carol E., Jason F. Arnold, and Judith C. Ahronheim, "Refusing Artificial Nutrition and Hydration: Does Statutory Law Send the Wrong Message?" Journal of the American Geriatrics Society 50, no. 3 (2002): 544–50.

## PART TWO: GUIDELINES ON CARE PLANNING AND DECISION-MAKING

### Section 1: Guidelines for Advance Care Planning and Advance Directives

Brasic, Gerlyn M. and Bernard J. Hammes. "Can't We Improve on Advance Directives?" Annals of Internal Medicine 148, no. 5 (2008): 405–6; authors' reply, 406.

Briggs, Linda A., Karin T. Kirchhoff, Bernard J. Hammes, Mi-Kyung Song, and Elaine R. Colvin. "Patient-centered Advance Care Planning in Special Patient Populations: A Pilot Study." Journal of Professional Nursing: Official Journal of the American Association of Colleges of Nursing 20, no. 1 (2004): 47–58.

Emanuel, Linda L. "Advance Care Planning for Decisional Incapacity: Keep It Simple—Find Your Patient's Goal Threshold in Under 5 Minutes." Medscape Journal of Medicine 10, no. 10 (2008): 240.

Fischer, Gary S., Hillel R. Alpert, John D. Stoeckle, and Linda L. Emanuel. "Can Goals of Care Be Used to Predict Intervention Preferences in an Advance Directive?" Archives of Internal Medicine 157, no. 7 (1997): 801–7.

Furman, Christian Davis, Susan E. Kelly, Keith Knapp, Robyn L. Mowery, and Toni Miles. "Eliciting Goals of Care in a Nursing Home." Journal of the American Medical Directors Association 8, no. 3, suppl. 2 (2007): e35–41.

Hammes, Bernard J., Judy Klevan, Michelle Kempf, and Marc S. Williams. "Pediatric Advance Care Planning." Journal of Palliative Medicine 8, no. 4 (2005): 766–73.

Hammes, Bernard J., and Brenda L. Rooney. "Death and End-of-Life Planning in One Midwestern Community." Archives of Internal Medicine 158, no. 4 (1998): 383–90.

Lynn, Joanne, and Nathan E. Goldstein. "Advance Care Planning for Fatal Chronic Illness: Avoiding Commonplace Errors and Unwarranted Suffering." Annals of Internal Medicine 138, no. 10 (2003): 812–18.

Romer, Anna L., and Bernard J. Hammes. "Communication, Trust, and Making Choices: Advance Care Planning Four Years On." Journal of Palliative Medicine 7, no. 2 (2004): 335–40.

Winter, Laraine, Susan M. Parks, and James J. Diamond. "Ask a Different Question, Get a Different Answer: Why Living Wills Are Poor Guides to Care Preferences at the End of Life." Journal of Palliative Medicine 13, no. 5 (2010): 567–72.

Wolf, Susan M., Philip Boyle, Daniel Callahan, Joseph J. Fins, Bruce Jennings, James Lindemann Nelson, Jeremiah A. Barondess, Dan W. Brock, Rebecca Dresser, Linda Emanuel, Sandra Johnson, John Lantos, DaCosta R. Mason, Mathy Mezey, David Orentlicher, and Fenella Rouse. "Sources of Concern About the Patient Self-Determination Act." NEJM 325 (1991): 1666–71.

### Section 2: Guidelines for the Decision-Making Process

Appelbaum, Paul S. "Assessment of Patients' Competence to Consent to Treatment." NEJM 357 (2007):1834–40.

Cantor, Norman L. "The Bane of Surrogate Decision Making: Defining the Best Interests of Never-Competent Persons." Journal of Legal Medicine 26, no. 2 (2005): 155–205.

Dresser, Rebecca S., and John A. Robertson. "Quality of Life and Non-Treatment Decisions for Incompetent Patients: A Critique of the Orthodox Approach." Journal of Law, Medicine & Ethics 17, no. 3 (1989): 234–44.

Gehlbach, Thomas G., Laura A. Shinkunas, Valeria L. Forman-Hoffman, Karl W. Thomas, Gregory A. Schmidt, and Lauris C. Kaldjian. "Code Status Orders and Goals of Care in the Medical ICU." Chest 139, no. 4 (2011): 802–9.

Hirschman, Karen B., Colette M. Joyce, Bryan D. James, Sharon X. Xie, and Jason H.T. Karlawish. "Do Alzheimer's Disease Patients Want to Participate in a Treatment Decision, and Would Their Caregivers Let Them?" Gerontologist 45, no. 3 (2005): 381–88.

Karlawish, Jason H.T., Timothy E. Quill, and Diane E. Meier. "A Consensus-Based Approach to Providing Palliative Care to Patients who Lack Decision-Making Capacity. ACP-ASIM End-of-Life Care Consensus Panel. American College of Physicians-American Society of Internal Medicine." Annals of Internal Medicine 130, no. 10 (1999): 835–40.

Karp, Naomi, and Erica Wood. *Incapacitated and Alone: Healthcare Decision-Making for the Unbefriended Elderly.* Washington, DC: ABA Commission on Law and Aging, 2003.

Kim, Scott Y.H., Jason Karlawish, H. Myra Kim, Ian F. Wall, Andrea C. Bozoki, and Paul S. Appelbaum. "Preservation of the Capacity to Appoint a Proxy Decision Maker: Implications for Dementia Research." Archives of General Psychiatry 68, no. 2 (2011): 214–20.

Meisel, Alan, and Mark Kuczewski. "Legal and Ethical Myths about Informed Consent." Archives of Internal Medicine 156, no. 22 (1996): 2521–26.

Quill, Timothy E., Robert Arnold, and Anthony L. Back. "Discussing Treatment Preferences with Patients Who Want 'Everything.'" Annals of Internal Medicine 151, no. 5 (2009): 345–49.

Sulmasy, Daniel P., and Lois Snyder. "Substituted Interests and Best Judgments: An Integrated Model of Surrogate Decision-Making." JAMA 304, no. 17 (2010): 1946–47.

Veterans Health Administration, VHA Handbook 1004.01. *Informed Consent for Clinical Treatments and Procedures* (effective August 17, 2009). Available at: http://www.va.gov/vhapublications/.

Wendler, David, and Annette Rid. "Can We Improve Decision-Making for Incapacitated Patients?" Hastings Center Report 40, no. 5 (2010): 36–45.

———. "Systematic Review: The Effect on Surrogates of Making Treatment Decisions for Others." Annals of Internal Medicine 154, no. 5 (2011): 336–46.

White, Douglas B., J. Randall Curtis, Leslie E. Wolf, Thomas J. Prendergast, Darren B. Taichman, Gary Kuniyoshi, Frank Acerra, Bernard Lo, and John M. Luce. "Life Support for Patients Without a Surrogate Decision Maker: Who Decides?" Annals of Internal Medicine 147, no. 1 (2007): 34–40.

### Section 3: Guidelines Concerning Neonates, Infants, Children and Adolescents

**Communication and collaboration with pediatric patients and surrogates**

Barfield, Raymond C., Debra Brandon, Julie Thompson, Nichol Harris, Michael Schmidt, and Sharron Docherty. "Mind the Child: Using Interactive Technology to Improve Child Involvement in Decision-Making About Life-Limiting Illness." American Journal of Bioethics 10, no. 4 (2010): 28–30.

Feudtner, Chris. "Collaborative Communication in Pediatric Palliative Care: A Foundation for Problem-Solving and Decision-Making." Pediatric Clinics of North America 54, no. 5 (2007): 583–607.

Hardart, George. "Including the Family's Interests in Medical Decision Making in Pediatrics." Journal of Clinical Ethics 11, no. 2 (2000): 164–68.

Heller, Karen S., and Mildred Z. Solomon. "Continuity of Caring: What Matters to Parents of Children with Life-Threatening Conditions." Journal of Pediatric Nursing 20, no. 5 (2005): 335–46.

Levetown, Marcia. "Communicating with Children and Families: From Everyday Interactions to Skill in Conveying Distressing Information." Pediatrics 121, no. 5 (2008): e1441–60.

Mack, Jennifer W., and Holcombe E. Grier. "The Day One Talk." Journal of Clinical Oncology 22, no. 3 (2004): 563–66.

Ross, Lainie Friedman. "Why 'Doctor, If This Were Your Child, What Would You Do?' Deserves an Answer." Journal of Clinical Ethics 14, nos. 1–2 (2003): 59–62. See also: Robert Truog. "Response." Journal of Clinical Ethics 14, nos. 1–2 (2003): 63–67; William Ruddick. "Response." Journal of Clinical Ethics 14, nos. 1–2 (2003): 68–70; and Jodi Halpern. "Response." Journal of Clinical Ethics 14, nos. 1–2 (2003): 71–78.

Sharman, Mahesh, Kathleen L. Meert, and Ashok P. Sarnaik. "What Influences Parents' Decisions to Limit or Withdraw Life Support?" Pediatric Critical Care Medicine 6, no. 5 (2005): 513–18.

**Assent, dissent, permission, consent, and refusal involving pediatric patients**

American Academy of Pediatrics Committee on Bioethics. "Informed Consent, Parental Permission, and Assent in Pediatric Practice." Pediatrics 95, no. 2 (1995): 314–17. Reaffirmed 2007.

——— and Committee on School Health. "Honoring Do-Not-Attempt-Resuscitation Requests in Schools." Pediatrics 125, no. 5 (2010): 1073–77.

Badzek, Laurie, and Sherry Kanosky. "Mature Minors and End-of-Life Decision-Making: A New Development in Their Legal Right to Participation." Journal of Nursing Law 8, no. 3 (2002): 23–29.

Halpern-Felsher, Bonnie L., and Elizabeth Cauffman. "Costs and Benefits of a Decision: Decision-Making Competence in Adolescents and Adults." Journal of Applied Developmental Psychology 22, no. 3 (2001): 257–73.

Mercurio, Mark R. "An Adolescent's Refusal of Medical Treatment: Implications of the Abraham Cheerix Case." Pediatrics 120, no. 6 (2007): 1357–58.

Miller, Victoria A., Dennis Drotar, and Eric Kodish. "Children's Competence for Assent and Consent: A Review of Empirical Findings." Ethics and Behavior 14, no. 3 (2004): 255–95.

Shaddy, Robert E., Scott C. Denne, and the Committee on Drugs and Committee on Pediatric Research of the American Academy of Pediatrics. "Guidelines for the Ethical Conduct of Studies to Evaluate Drugs in Pediatrics Populations." Pediatrics 125, no. 4 (2010): 850–60.

### Treatment decision-making concerning neonates

American Academy of Pediatrics. "Clinical Report: Antenatal Counseling Regarding Resuscitation at an Extremely Low Gestational Age." Pediatrics 124, no. 1 (2009): 422–27.

Annas, George J. "Extremely Preterm Birth and Parental Authority to Refuse Treatment: The Case of Sidney Miller." NEJM 351, no. 20 (2004): 2118–22.

Janvier, Annie, Karen Lynn Bauer, and John D. Lantos. "Are Newborns Morally Different from Older Children?" Theoretical Medicine and Bioethics 28 (2007): 413–25.

Lantos, John D., and William L. Meadow. Neonatal Bioethics: The Moral Challenges of Medical Innovation. Baltimore, MD: Johns Hopkins University Press, 2006.

MacDonald, Hugh, and the Committee on Fetus and Newborn, "Perinatal Care at the Threshold of Viability," Pediatrics 110, no. 5 (2002): 1024–27.

Mercurio, Mark R. "The Ethics of Newborn Resuscitation." Seminars in Perinatology 33, no. 6 (2009): 354–63.

Pignotti, Maria Serenella, and Gianpaolo Donzelli. "Perinatal Care at the Threshold of Viability: An International Comparison of Practical Guidelines for the Treatment of Extremely Preterm Births." Pediatrics 121, no. 1 (2008): e193–98.

Tyson, Jon E., Nehal A. Parikh, John Langer, Charles Green, and Rosemary D. Higgins. "Intensive Care for Extreme Prematurity—Moving beyond Gestational Age." NEJM 358, no. 16 (2008): 1672–81.

### Treatment decision-making and end-of-life care

American Academy of Pediatrics Committee on Bioethics. "Ethics and the Care of Critically Ill Infants and Children." Pediatrics 98, no. 1 (1996): 149–52.

———. "Guidelines on Foregoing Life-Sustaining Medical Treatment." Pediatrics 93, no. 3 (1994): 532–36. Reaffirmed 2009.

Burns, Jeffrey P., Christine Mitchell, John L. Griffith, and Robert D. Truog. "End-of-Life Care in the Pediatric Intensive Care Unit: Attitudes and Practices of Pediatric Critical Care Physicians and Nurses." Critical Care Medicine 29, no. 3 (2001): 658–64.

National Hospice and Palliative Care Organization. Standards for Pediatric Palliative and Hospice Care: Advancing Care for America's Children. Alexandria, VA: National Hospice and Palliative Care Organization, 2009.

Solomon, Mildred Z., Deborah Sellers, Karen Heller, Deborah Dokken, Marcia Levetown, Cynda Rushton, Robert D. Truog, and Alan Fleischman. "New and Lingering Controversies in Pediatric End-of-Life Care." Pediatrics 116, no. 4 (2005): 872–83.

Weiner, Julie, Jotishna Sharma, John Lantos, and Howard Kilbride. "How Infants Die in the Neonatal Intensive Care Unit: Trends from 1999 through 2008." Archives of Pediatric and Adolescent Medicine 165, no. 7 (2011): 630–34.

Wolf, Susan M. "Facing Assisted Suicide and Euthanasia in Children and Adolescents." In: Regulating How We Die: The Ethical, Medical, and Legal Issues Surrounding Physician-Assisted Suicide, ed. Linda L. Emanuel. Cambridge, MA: Harvard University Press, 1998.

### Surrogate decision-making for abused children

American Academy of Pediatrics Committee on Bioethics and Committee on Child Abuse and Neglect. "Forgoing Life-Sustaining Medical Treatment in Abused Children." Pediatrics 106, no. 5 (2000): 1151–53.

Gladsjo, Julie Akiko, John Breding, David Sine, Robert Wells, Sharon Kalemkiarian, Joni Oak, Angela S. Vieira, and Sheila Fallo Friedlander. "Termination of Life Support after Severe Child Abuse: The Role of a Guardian ad Litem." Pediatrics 113, no. 2 (2004): e141–45.

218    SELECTED BIBLIOGRAPHY

*Section 4: Guidelines for Care Transitions*

**Hand-offs between professionals**

Arora, Vineet, Sandeep Gangireddy, Amit Mehrotra, Ranjan Ginde, Megan Tormey, and David Meltzer. "Ability of Hospitalized Patients to Identify Their In-Hospital Physicians." Archives of Internal Medicine 169, no. 2 (2009): 199–201.

Arora, Vineet M., Efren Manjarrez, Daniel D. Dressler, Preetha Basaviah, Lakshmi Halasyamani, and Sunil Kripalani. "Hospitalist Handoffs: A Systematic Review and Task Force Recommendations." Journal of Hospital Medicine 4, no. 7 (2009): 433–40.

Kuo, Yong-Fang, Gulshan Sharma, Jean L. Freeman, and James S. Goodwin. "Growth in the Care of Older Patients by Hospitalists in the United States." NEJM 360, no. 11 (2009): 1102–12.

Vidyarthi, Arpana R., Vineet Arora, Jeffrey L. Schnipper, Susan D. Wall, and Robert M. Wachter. "Managing Discontinuity in Academic Medical Centers: Strategies for a Safe and Effective Resident Sign-Out." Journal of Hospital Medicine 1, no. 4 (2006): 257–66.

Welsh, Catherine Amber, Mindy E. Flanagan, and Patricia Ebright. "Barriers and Facilitators to Nursing Handoffs: Recommendations for Redesign." Nursing Outlook 58, no. 3 (2010): 148–54.

**Care transitions for nursing home residents**

Boockvar, Kenneth, Eliot Fishman, Corinne Kay Kyriacou, Anna Monias, Shai Gavi, and Tara Cortes. "Adverse Events Due to Discontinuations in Drug Use and Dose Changes in Patients Transferred Between Acute and Long-Term Care Facilities." Archives of Internal Medicine 164, no. 5 (2004): 545–50.

Casarett, David, Jason Karlawish, Knashawn Morales, Roxane Crowley, Terre Mirsch, and David A. Asch. "Improving the Use of Hospice Services in Nursing Homes: A Randomized Controlled Trial." JAMA 294, no. 2 (2005): 211–17.

Center to Advance Palliative Care. *Improving Palliative Care in Nursing Homes*. New York: Center to Advance Palliative Care, 2007.

Gessert, Charles E., Barbara Elliott, and Cynthia Peden-McAlpine. "Family Decision-Making for Nursing Home Residents with Dementia: Rural-Urban Differences." Journal of Rural Health 22, no. 1 (2006): 1–8.

Gozalo, Pedro, Joan M. Teno, Susan L. Mitchell, Jon Skinner, Julie Bynum, Denise Tyler, and Vincent Mor. "End-of-Life Transitions among Nursing Home Residents with Cognitive Issues." NEJM 365, no. 13 (2011): 1212–21.

Johnson, Sandra. "Living and Dying in Nursing Homes," In: *Ethical Dilemmas at the End of Life*, ed. Kenneth Doka, Bruce Jennings, and Charles Corr. Washington, DC: Hospice Foundation of America, 2005.

Kapp, Marshall B. "Legal Anxieties and End-of-Life Care in Nursing Homes." Issues in Law and Medicine 19, no. 2 (2003): 111–34.

Miller, Susan C., and Beth Han. "End-of-Life Care in U.S. Nursing Homes: Nursing Homes with Special Programs and Trained Staff for Hospice or Palliative/End-of-Life Care." Journal of Palliative Medicine 11, no. 6 (2008): 866–77.

Mitchell, Susan L., Joan M. Teno, Dan K. Kiely, Michele L. Shaffer, Richard N. Jones, Holly G. Prigerson, Ladislav Volicer, Jane L. Givens, and Mary Beth Hamel. "The Clinical Course of Advanced Dementia." NEJM 361, no. 16 (2009): 1529–38.

Mor, Vincent, Orna Intrator, Zhanlian Feng, and David C. Grabowski. "The Revolving Door of Rehospitalization from Skilled Nursing Facilities." Health Affairs 29, no. 1 (2010): 57–64.

Parker-Oliver, Debra, and Denise Bickel. "Nursing Home Experience with Hospice." Journal of the American Medical Directors Association 3, no. 2 (2002): 46–50.

Sloane, Philip D., Sheryl Zimmerman, Laura Hanson, C. Madeline Mitchell, Charlene Riedel-Leo, and Verita Custis-Buie. "End-of-Life Care in Assisted Living and Related Residential Care Settings." Journal of the American Geriatrics Society 51, no. 11 (2003): 1587–94.

Tilly, Jane, Peter Reed, Elizabeth Gould, and Abel Fok. *Dementia Care Practice: Recommendations for Assisted Living Residences and Nursing Homes, Phase 3: End-of-Life Care*. Chicago, IL: Alzheimer's Association, 2007.

**Use of CPR in nursing homes**

Applebaum, Gary E., Joyce E. King, and Thomas E. Finucane. "The Outcome of CPR Initiated in Nursing Homes." Journal of the American Geriatrics Society 38, no. 3 (1990): 197–200.

Sasson, Camilla, Mary A.M. Rogers, Jason Dahl, and Arthur L. Kellermann. "Predictors of Survival from Out-of-Hospital Cardiac Arrest: A Systematic Review and Meta-Analysis." Circulation: Cardiovascular Quality and Outcomes 3, no. 1 (2010): 63–81.

Shah, Manish N., Rollin J. Fairbanks, and E. Brooke Lerner. "Cardiac Arrests in Skilled Nursing Facilities: Continuing Room for Improvement." Journal of the American Medical Directors Association 8, no. 3, suppl. 2 (2007): e27–31.

## Use of feeding tubes in nursing homes

Lopez, Ruth Palan, Elaine J. Amella, Neville E. Strumpf, Joan M. Teno, and Susan L. Mitchell. "The Influence of Nursing Home Culture on the Use of Feeding Tubes." Archives of Internal Medicine 170, no. 1 (2010): 83–88.

Teno, Joan M, Susan L. Mitchell, Sylvia K. Kuo, Pedro L. Gozalo, Ramona L. Rhodes, Julie C. Lima, and Vincent Mor. "Decision-Making and Outcomes of Feeding Tube Insertion: A Five-State Study." Journal of the American Geriatrics Society 59, no. 5 (2011): 881–86.

Teno, Joan M, Susan L. Mitchell, Jonathan Skinner, Sylvia Kuo, Elliott Fisher, Orna Intrator, Ramona Rhodes, and Vincent Mor. "Churning: The Association between Health Care Transitions and Feeding Tube Insertion for Nursing Home Residents with Advanced Cognitive Impairment." Journal of Palliative Medicine 12, no. 4 (2009): 359–62.

## Portable medical orders/POLST

Hickman, Susan E., Christine A. Nelson, Nancy A. Perrin, Alvin H. Moss, Bernard J. Hammes, and Susan W. Tolle. "A Comparison of Methods to Communicate Treatment Preferences in Nursing Facilities: Traditional Practices Versus the Physician Orders for Life-Sustaining Treatment Program." Journal of the American Geriatrics Society 58, no. 7 (2010): 1241–48.

Hickman, Susan E., Susan W. Tolle, Kenneth Brummel-Smith, and Margaret Murphy Carley. "Use of the Physician Orders for Life-Sustaining Treatment Program in Oregon Nursing Facilities: Beyond Resuscitation Status." Journal of the American Geriatrics Society 52, no. 9 (2004): 1424–29.

Schmidt, Terri, Susan E. Hickman, Susan W. Tolle, and Heather S. Brooks. "The Physician Orders for Life-Sustaining Treatment Program: Oregon Emergency Medical Technicians' Practical Experiences and Attitudes." Journal of the American Geriatrics Society 52, no. 9 (2004): 1430–34.

## Discharge planning

Forster, Alan J., Harvey J. Murff, Josh F. Peterson, Tejal K. Gandhi, and David W. Bates. "The Incidence and Severity of Adverse Events Affecting Patients after Discharge from the Hospital." Annals of Internal Medicine 138, no. 3 (2003): 161–67.

Kripalani, Sunil, Amy T. Jackson, Jeffrey L. Schnipper, and Eric A Coleman. "Promoting Effective Transitions of Care at Hospital Discharge: A Review of Key Issues for Hospitalists." Journal of Hospital Medicine 2, no. 5 (2007): 314–23.

Kripalani, Sunil, Frank LeFevre, Christopher O. Phillips, Mark V. Williams, Preetha Basaviah, and David W. Baker. "Deficits in Communication and Information Transfer between Hospital-Based and Primary Care Physicians: Implications for Patient Safety and Continuity of Care." JAMA 297, no. 8 (2007): 831–41.

Mitnick, Sheryl, Cathy Leffler, and Virginia L. Hood, for the American College of Physicians Ethics, Professionalism and Human Rights Committee. "Family Caregivers, Patients and Physicians: Ethical Guidance to Optimize Relationships." Journal of General Internal Medicine 25, no. 3 (2010): 255–60.

Were, Martin C., Xiaochun Li, Joe Kesterson, Jason Cadwallader, Chite Asirwa, Babar Khan, and Marc B. Rosenman. "Adequacy of Hospital Discharge Summaries in Documenting Tests with Pending Results and Outpatient Follow-Up Providers." Journal of General Internal Medicine 24, no. 9 (2009): 1002–1006.

## End-of-life care in the hospital

Barbera, Lisa, Carole Taylor, and Deborah Dudgeon. "Why Do Patients Visit the Emergency Department Near the End of Life?" Canadian Medical Association Journal 182, no. 6 (2010): 563–68.

Lamba, Sangeeta, and Tammie E. Quest. "Hospice Care and the Emergency Department: Rules, Regulations, and Referrals." Annals of Emergency Medicine 57, no. 3 (2011): 282–90.

Miller, Franklin G., and Joseph J. Fins. "A Proposal to Restructure Hospital Care for Dying Patients." NEJM 334 (1996): 1740–42.

Smith, Alexander K., Jonathan Fisher, Mara A. Shonberg, Daniel J. Pallin, Susan D. Block, Lachlan Forrow, Russell S. Phillips, and Ellen P. McCarthy. "Am I Doing the Right Thing? Provider Perspectives on Improving Palliative Care in the Emergency Department." Annals of Emergency Medicine 54, no. 1 (2009): 86–93.

*Section 5: Guidelines for the Determination of Death*

Ad Hoc Committee of the Harvard Medical School to Examine the Definition of Brain Death. "A Definition of Irreversible Coma." JAMA 205, no. 6 (1968): 337–40.

Applbaum, Arthur Isak, Jon C. Tilburt, Michael T. Collins, and David Wendler. "A Family's Request for Complementary Medicine after Patient Brain Death." JAMA 299, no. 18 (2008): 2188–93. See also: Kompanje, Erwin J.O. "Request for Complementary Medicine after Brain Death." JAMA 300, no. 13 (2008): 1517; McCullough, Laurence B. "Request for Complementary Medicine after Brain Death." JAMA 300, no. 13 (2008): 1517; and Applbaum, Arthur Isak, and Jon C. Tilbert. "Request for Complementary Medicine after Brain Death—Reply." JAMA 300, no. 13 (2008): 1517–18.

Capron, Alexander M. and Fred H. Cate. "Death and Organ Donation." In: *Treatise on Health Care Law*, ed. Matthew Bender. New York: Matthew Bender, 1991.

Capron, Alexander M., and Leon R. Kass. "A Statutory Definition of the Standards for Determining Human Death." University of Pennsylvania Law Review 121 (1972): 87–118.

Cate, Fred H. "Human Organ and Tissue Transplantation: The Role of Law." Journal of Corporation Law 20 (1994): 69–90.

Lammers, Stephen E., Lauren B. Smith, and Patricia J. Lyndale. "Too Much to Ask?" Hastings Center Report 41, no. 4 (2011): 15–16.

President's Commission for the Study of Ethical Problems in Medicine and Biomedical and Behavioral Research. *Defining Death: Medical, Legal and Ethical Issues in the Determination of Death*. Washington, DC: U.S. Government Printing Office, 1981.

Wijdicks, Eelco F.M., Panayiotis N. Varelas, Gary S. Gronseth, and David M. Greer. "Evidence-Based Guideline Update: Determining Brain Death in Adults." Neurology 74, no. 23 (2010): 1911–18.

**Donation after cardiac death**

Bernat, James L. "The Boundaries of Organ Donation after Circulatory Death." NEJM 359, no. 7 (2008): 669–71.

Boucek, Mark M., Christine Mashburn, Susan Dunn, Rebecca Frizell, Leah Edwards, Biagio Pietra, and David Campbell. "Pediatric Heart Transplantation after Declaration of Cardiac Death." NEJM 359, no. 7 (2008): 709–14.

Solomon, Mildred Z. "Maximizing Benefits, Minimizing Harms: A Research Agenda to Assess the Impact of Non-Heart-Beating Organ Donation." In: Committee on Non-Heart-Beating Transplantation II: The Scientific and Ethical Basis for Practice and Protocols, Division of Health Care Services, Institute of Medicine. *Non-Heart-Beating Organ Transplantation: Practice and Protocols*. Washington, DC: National Academy of Science, 2000.

Truog, Robert, and Franklin G. Miller. "The Dead Donor Rule and Organ Transplantation." NEJM 359, no. 7 (2008): 674–75.

Veatch, Robert M. "Donating Hearts after Cardiac Death: Reversing the Irreversible." NEJM 359 no. 7 (2008): 672–73.

Youngner, Stuart J., Robert M. Arnold, and Renie Schapiro, eds. *The Definition of Death: Contemporary Controversies*. Baltimore, MD: Johns Hopkins University Press, 1999.

*Section 6: Guidelines for Institutional Policy*

**Ethics services, including ethics committees and clinical ethics consultation**

American Society for Bioethics and Humanities. *Core Competencies for Health Care Ethics Consultation*. 2d ed. Glenview, IL: American Society for Bioethics and Humanities, 2011.

Berkowitz, Kenneth, and Nancy N. Dubler. "Approaches to Ethics Consultations." In: *Handbook for Healthcare Ethics Committees*, ed. Linda Farber Post, Jeffrey Blustein, and Nancy N. Dubler, Baltimore, MD: Johns Hopkins University Press, 2007.

Dubler, Nancy N., Mayris P. Webber, and Deborah M. Swiderski. "Charting the Future: Credentialing, Privileging, Quality, and Evaluation in Clinical Ethics Consultation." Hastings Center Report 39, no. 6 (2009): 23–33.

Fox, Ellen, Sarah Myers, and Robert A. Pearlman. "Ethics Consultation in United States Hospitals: A National Survey." American Journal of Bioethics 7, no. 2 (2007): 13–25.

Powell, Tia, and Jeffrey Blustein. "Introduction: The Nature and Functioning of Ethics Committees." In: *Handbook for Healthcare Ethics Committees*, ed. Linda Farber Post, Jeffrey Blustein, and Nancy N. Dubler, Baltimore, MD: Johns Hopkins University Press, 2007.

Solomon, Mildred Z., Bruce Jennings, Vivian Guilfoy, Rebecca Jackson, Lydia O'Donnell, Susan M. Wolf, Kathleen Nolan, Dieter Koch-Weser, and Strachan Donnelley. "Toward an Expanded Vision of Clinical Ethics Education: From the Individual to the Institution." Kennedy Institute of Ethics Journal 1 (1991): 225–45.

Wolf, Susan M. "Ethics Committees and Due Process: Nesting Rights in a Community of Caring." Maryland Law Review 50 (1991): 798–858.

### Palliative care services

Cintron, Alexie, and R. Sean Morrison. "Pain and Ethnicity in the United States: A Systematic Review." Journal of Palliative Medicine 9, no. 6 (2006): 1454–73.

Goldsmith, Benjamin, Jessica Dietrich, Qingling Du, and R. Sean Morrison. "Variability in Access to Hospital Palliative Care in the United States." Journal of Palliative Medicine 11, no. 8 (2008): 1094–1102.

Lynn, Joanne, Marie W. Schall, Casey Milne, Kevin M. Nolan, and Andrea Kabcenell, "Quality Improvements in End of Life Care: Insights from Two Collaboratives." Joint Commission Journal on Quality Improvement 26, no. 5 (2000): 254–67.

Morrison, R. Sean, Joan D. Penrod, J. Brian Cassel, Melissa Caust-Ellenbogen, Ann Litke, Lynn Spragens, and Diane E. Meier, for the Palliative Care Leadership Centers' Outcomes Group. "Cost Savings Associated with U.S. Hospital Palliative Care Consultation Programs." Archives of Internal Medicine 168, no. 16, (2008): 1783–90.

National Rural Health Association. *Providing Hospice and Palliative Care in Rural and Frontier Areas*. Kansas City, MO: National Rural Health Association, 2006.

Rich, Shayna E., Ann L. Gruber-Baldini, Charlene C. Quinn, and Sheryl I. Zimmerman. "Discussion as a Factor in Racial Disparity in Advance Directive Completion at Nursing Home Admission." Journal of the American Geriatrics Society 57, no. 1 (2009): 146–52.

Weissman, David E., and Diane E. Meier. "Identifying Patients in Need of a Palliative Care Assessment in the Hospital Setting," Journal of Palliative Medicine 14, no. 1, special report (2011): 1–7.

### Advance care planning

Degenholtz, Howard B., Robert A. Arnold, Alan Meisel, and Judith R. Lave. "Persistence of Racial Disparities in Advance Care Plan Documents Among Nursing Home Residents." Journal of the American Geriatrics Society 50, no. 2 (2002): 378–81.

Smith, Alexander K., Ellen P. McCarthy, Elizabeth Paulk, Tracy A. Balboni, Paul K. Maciejewski, Susan D. Block, and Holly G. Prigerson. "Racial and Ethnic Differences in Advance Care Planning Among Patients with Cancer: Impact of Terminal Illness Acknowledgment, Religiousness, and Treatment Preferences." Journal of Clinical Oncology 26, no. 25 (2008): 4131–37.

### Portable medical orders: Policy

Hickman, Susan E., Charles P. Sabatino, Alvin H. Moss, and Jessica Wehrle Nester. "The POLST (Physician Orders for Life-Sustaining Treatment) Paradigm to Improve End-of-Life Care: Potential State Legal Barriers to Implementation." Journal of Law, Medicine & Ethics 36, no.1 (2008): 119–40.

### Care transitions: Policy

Finucane, Thomas E., and G. Michael Harper. "Attempting Resuscitation in Nursing Homes: Policy Considerations." Journal of the American Geriatrics Society 47, no. 10 (1999): 1261–64.

Hoffman, Diane E., and Anita J. Tarzian. "Dying in America: An Examination of Policies That Deter Adequate End-of-Life Care in Nursing Homes." Journal of Law, Medicine & Ethics 33, no. 2 (2005): 294–309.

O'Mahoney, Sean, Janet McHenry, Daniel Snow, Carolyn Cassin, Donald Schumacher, and Peter A. Selwyn. "A Review of Barriers to Utilization of the Medicare Hospice Benefits in Urban Populations and Strategies for Enhanced Access." Journal of Urban Health 85, no. 2 (2008): 281–90.

Perry, Shawna J., Robert L. Wears, and Emily S. Patterson. "High-Hanging Fruit: Improving Transitions in Health Care." In: *Advances in Patient Safety: New Directions and Alternative Approaches, Volume 3: Performance and Tools*, ed. Kerm Henriksen, James B. Battles, Eric S. Marks, and David I. Lewis. Rockville, MD: Agency for Healthcare Research and Quality, 2008.

**Legal counsel and risk management**

Sabatino, Charles P. "The Evolution of Health Care Advance Planning Law and Policy." Milbank Quarterly 88, no. 2 (2010): 211–39.

Spear, Steven J., and Mark Schmidhofer. "Ambiguity and Workarounds as Contributors to Medical Error." Annals of Internal Medicine 142, no. 8 (2005): 627–30.

Zuckerman, Connie. *End-of-Life Care and Hospital Legal Counsel: Current Involvement and Opportunities for the Future*. New York: United Hospital Fund and Milbank Memorial Fund, 1999.

**Conflict resolution**

Dubler, Nancy N., and Carol B. Liebman. *Bioethics Mediation: A Guide to Shaping Shared Solutions*. Rev. ed. Nashville, TN: Vanderbilt University Press/United Hospital Fund, 2011.

Pope, Thaddeus Mason. "Legal Briefing: Conscience Clauses and Conscientious Refusal." Journal of Clinical Ethics 21, no. 2 (2010): 163–80.

Wicclair, Mark R. *Conscientious Objection in Health Care: An Ethical Analysis*. New York: Cambridge University Press, 2011.

## PART THREE: COMMUNICATION SUPPORTING DECISION-MAKING AND CARE

*Section 1: Communication with Patients, Surrogates, and Loved Ones*

Casarett, David, Amy Pickard, Jessica M. Fishman, Stewart C. Alexander, Robert M. Arnold, Kathryn I. Pollack, and James A. Tulsky. "Can Metaphors and Analogies Improve Communication with Seriously Ill Patients?" Journal of Palliative Medicine 13, no. 3 (2010): 255–60.

Curtis, J. Randall, Donald L. Patrick, Sarah E. Shannon, Patsy D. Treece, Ruth A. Engelberg, and Gordon D. Rubenfeld. "The Family Conference as a Focus to Improve Communication about End-of-Life Care in the Intensive Care Unit: Opportunities for Improvement." Critical Care Medicine 29, no. 2, suppl. (2001): N26–33.

Goldstein, Nathan E., Anthony L. Back, and Sean R. Morrison. "Titrating Guidance: A Model to Guide Physicians in Assisting Patients and Family Members Who Are Facing Complex Decisions." Archives of Internal Medicine 168, no. 16 (2008): 1733–39.

Teno, Joan M., Brian R. Clarridge, Virginia Casey, Lisa C. Welch, Terrie Wetle, Renee Shield, and Vincent Mor. "Family Perspectives on End-of-Life Care at the Last Place of Care." JAMA 91, no. 1 (2004): 88–93.

Tulsky, James A. "Beyond Advance Directives: Importance of Communication Skills at the End of Life." JAMA 294, no. 3 (2005): 359–65.

*Section 2: Communication and Collaboration with Patients with Disabilities*

Cea, Christine D., and Celia B. Fisher. "Health Care Decision Making by Adults with Mental Retardation." Mental Retardation 41, no. 2 (2003): 78–87.

Ferguson, Morag, Dominic Jarrett, and Melody Terras. "Inclusion and Healthcare Choices: The Experiences of Adults with Learning Disabilities." British Journal of Learning Disabilities 39, no. 1 (2011): 73–83.

Friedman, Sandra L., and David T. Helm, eds. *End-of-Life Care for Children and Adults with Intellectual and Developmental Disabilities*. Washington, DC: American Association on Intellectual and Developmental Disabilities, 2010.

Ganzini, Linda, Ladislav Volicer, William A. Nelson, Ellen Fox, and Arthur R. Derse. "Ten Myths about Decision-Making Capacity." Journal of the American Medical Directors Association 5, no. 4 (2004): 263–67.

The Hastings Center. "Summary Document," Guidelines project consultation with representatives of disability communities, convened by the Donnelley Ethics Program (formerly the Donnelley Family Disability Ethics Program) at the Rehabilitation Institute of Chicago, July 23–24, 2007 (unpublished working paper).

Kirschner, Kristi L. "Calling It Quits: When Patients or Proxies Request to Withdraw or Withhold Life-Sustaining Treatment after Spinal Cord Injury." Topics in Spinal Cord Injury Rehabilitation 13, no. 3 (2008): 30–43.

Kothari, Sunil, and Kristi L. Kirschner. "Abandoning the Golden Rule: The Problem with 'Putting Ourselves in the Patient's Place.'" Topics in Stroke Rehabilitation 13, no. 4 (2006): 68–73.

Pollens, Robin. "Role of the Speech-Language Pathologist in Palliative Hospice Care." Journal of Palliative Medicine 7, no. 5 (2004): 694–702.

Powell, Tia, and Bruce Lowenstein. "Refusing Life-Sustaining Treatment after Catastrophic Injury: Ethical Implications." Journal of Law, Medicine & Ethics 24, no. 1 (1996): 54–61.

Skinner, Rachael, Chris Joiner, Liz Chesters, Louise Bates, and Louise Scrivener. "Demystifying the Process? A Multi-Disciplinary Approach to Assessing Capacity for Adults with a Learning Disability." British Journal of Learning Disabilities 39, no. 2 (2011): 92–97.

*Section 3: Psychological Dimensions of Decision-Making about Life-Sustaining Treatment and Care Near the End of Life*

**Coping**

Block, Susan D. "Psychological Considerations, Growth, and Transcendence at the End of Life: The Art of the Possible." JAMA 285, no. 22 (2001): 2898–2905.

Boyd, Elizabeth A., Bernard Lo, Leah R. Evans, Grace Malvar, Latifat Apatira, John M. Luce, and Douglas B. White. "'It's Not Just What the Doctor Tells Me': Factors That Influence Surrogate Decision-Makers' Perceptions of Prognosis." Critical Care Medicine 38, no. 5 (2010): 1270–75.

Pearce, Michelle J., Jerome L. Singer, and Holly G. Prigerson. "Religious Coping among Caregivers of Terminally Ill Cancer Patients: Main Effects and Psychosocial Mediators." Journal of Health Psychology 11, no. 5 (2006): 743–59.

Phelps, Andrea C., Paul K. Maciejewski, Matthew Nilsson, Tracy A. Balboni, Alexi A. Wright, M. Elizabeth Paulk, Elizabeth Trice, Deborah Schrag, John R. Peteet, Susan D. Block, and Holly G. Prigerson. "Religious Coping and Use of Intensive Life-Prolonging Care Near Death in Patients with Advanced Cancer." JAMA 301, no. 11 (2009): 1140–47.

**Hope**

Jackson, Vicki A., Jennifer Mack, Robin Matsuyama, Mathew D. Lakoma, Amy M. Sullivan, Robert M. Arnold, Jane C. Weeks, and Susan D. Block. "A Qualitative Study of Oncologists' Approaches to End-of-Life Care." Journal of Palliative Medicine 11, no. 6 (2008): 893–906.

Quill, Timothy E., Robert M. Arnold, and Frederic Platt. "'I Wish Things Were Different': Expressing Wishes in Response to Loss, Futility, and Unrealistic Hopes." Annals of Internal Medicine 135, no. 7 (2001): 551–55.

Smith, Thomas J., Lindsay Dow, Enid Virago, James Khatcheressian, Laurel J. Lyckholm, and Robin Matsuyama. "Giving Honest Information to Patients with Advanced Cancer Maintains Hope." Oncology 24, no. 6 (2010): 521–25.

Steinhauser, Karen E. "Factors Considered Important at the End of Life by Patients, Family, Physicians, and Other Care Providers." JAMA 284, no. 19 (2000): 2476–82.

**Ambivalence, denial, and grief**

Maciejewski, Paul K., Baohui Zhang, Susan D. Block, and Holly G. Prigerson. "An Empirical Examination of the Stage Theory of Grief." JAMA 297, no. 7 (2007): 716–23.

Nilsson, Matthew E., Paul K. Maciejewski, Baohui Zhang, Alexi A. Wright, Elizabeth Trice, Anna C. Muriel, Robert J. Friedlander, Karen M. Fasciano, Susan D. Block, and Holly G. Prigerson. "Mental Health, Treatment Preferences, Advance Care Planning, and Location and Quality of Death in Advanced Cancer Patients with Dependent Children." Cancer 115, no. 2 (2009): 399–409.

Wright, Alexi A., Baohui Zhang, Alaka Ray, Jennifer W. Mack, Elizabeth Trice, Tracy Balboni, Susan L. Mitchell, Vicki A. Jackson, Susan D. Block, Paul K. Maciejewski, and Holly G. Prigerson. "Associations Between End-of-Life Discussions, Patient Mental Health, Medical Care Near Death, and Caregiver Bereavement Adjustment." JAMA 300, no. 14 (2008): 1665–73.

**Existential suffering**

Boston, Patricia, Anne Bruce, and Rita Schreiber. "Existential Suffering in the Palliative Care Setting: An Integrated Literature Review." Journal of Pain and Symptom Management 41, no. 3 (2011): 604–18.

Chochinov, Harvey M., Thomas Hassard, Susan McClement, Thomas Hack, Linda P. Kristjanson, Mike Harlos, Shane Sinclair, and Alison Murray. "The Landscape of Distress in the Terminally Ill." Journal of Pain and Symptom Management 38, no. 5 (2009): 641–49.

Lichtenthal, Wendy G., Matthew Nilsson, Baohui Zhang, Elizabeth D. Trice, David W. Kissane, William Breitbart, and Holly G. Prigerson. "Do Rates of Mental Disorders and Existential Distress among Advanced Stage Cancer Patients Increase as Death Approaches?" Psycho-Oncology 18, no. 1 (2009): 50–61.

## Spirituality and religion

Alcorn, Sara R., Michael J. Balboni, Holly G. Prigerson, Amy Reynolds, Andrea C. Phelps, Alexi A. Wright, Susan D. Block, John R. Peteet, Lisa A. Kachnic, and Tracy A. Balboni. "Provision of Spiritual Care to Patients with Advanced Cancer: Associations with Medical Care and Quality of Life Near Death." Journal of Clinical Oncology 28, no. 3 (2010): 445–52.

Puchalski, Christina, Betty Ferrell, Rose Virani, Shirley Otis-Green, Pamela Baird, Janet Bull, Harvey Chochinov, George Handzo, Holly Nelson-Becker, Maryjo Prince-Paul, Karen Pugliese, and Daniel Sulmasy. "Improving the Quality of Spiritual Care as a Dimension of Palliative Care." Journal of Palliative Medicine 12, no. 10 (2009): 885–904.

Robinson, Mary R., Mary M. Thiel, Meghan M. Backus, and Elaine C. Meyer. "Matters of Spirituality at the End of Life in the Pediatric Intensive Care Unit." Pediatrics 118, no. 3 (2006): e719–29.

Sulmasy, Daniel P. "Spiritual Issues in the Care of Dying Patients: '…It's Okay Between Me and God.'" JAMA 296, no. 11 (2006): 1385–92.

## Religious objections

American Academy of Pediatrics Committee on Bioethics. "Religious Objections to Medical Care." Pediatrics 99, no. 2 (1997): 279–81.

Fitchett, George. Assessing Spiritual Needs: A Guide for Caregivers. Minneapolis, MN: Augsburg Fortress, 1993.

Gillick, M. "Artificial Nutrition and Hydration in the Patient with Advanced Dementia: Is Withholding Treatment Compatible with Traditional Judaism?" Journal of Medical Ethics 27, no. 1 (2001): 12–15.

Gupta, Vidya B., and Debjani Mukherjee. "Conflicting Beliefs." Hastings Center Report 40, no. 4 (2010): 14–15.

Loike, John, Muriel Gillick, Stephan Mayer, Kenneth Prager, Jeremy R. Simon, Avraham Steinberg, Moshe D. Tendler, Mordechai Willig, and Ruth L. Fischbach. "The Critical Role of Religion: Caring for the Dying Patient from an Orthodox Jewish Perspective." Journal of Palliative Medicine 13, no. 10 (2010): 1267–71.

Puchalski, Christina, and Anna L. Romer. "Taking Spiritual History Allows Clinicians to Understand Patients More Fully." Journal of Palliative Medicine 3, no. 1 (2000): 129–37.

Steinhauser, Karen E., Corinne I. Voils, Elizabeth C. Clipp, Hayden B. Bosworth, Nicholas A. Christakis, and James A. Tulsky. "Are You at Peace? One Item to Probe Spiritual Concerns at the End of Life." Archives of Internal Medicine 166, no. 1 (2008): 101–5.

## Moral distress

Curtis, J. Randall, and Robert A. Burt. "Why Are Critical Care Clinicians So Powerfully Distressed by Family Demands for Futile Care?" Critical Care Medicine 18, no. 1 (2003): 22–24.

Epstein, Elizabeth G., and Ann B. Hamric. "Moral Distress, Moral Residue, and the Crescendo Effect." Journal of Clinical Ethics 20, no. 4 (2009): 330–42.

Ferrell, Betty R. "Understanding the Moral Distress of Nurses Witnessing Medically Futile Care." Oncology Nursing Forum 33, no. 5 (2006): 922–30.

Hamric, Ann B., and Leslie J. Blackhall. "Nurse-Physician Perspectives on the Care of Dying Patients in Intensive Care Units: Collaboration, Moral Distress, and Ethical Climate." Critical Care Medicine 35, no. 2 (2007): 422–29.

## Bereavement care

Kearney, Michael K., Radhule B. Weininger, Mary L.S. Vachon, Richard L. Harrison, and Balfour M. Mount. "Self-Care of Physicians Caring for Patients at the End of Life: 'Being Connected…A Key to My Survival.'" JAMA 301, no. 11 (2009): 1155–64.

Meier, Diane E., Anthony L. Back, and R. Sean Morrison. "The Inner Life of Physicians and Care of the Seriously Ill." JAMA 286, no. 23 (2001): 3007–14.

Smith, Alexander K., Mary K. Buss, David F. Giansiracusa, and Susan D. Block. "On Being Fired: Experiences of Patient-Initiated Termination of the Patient-Physician Relationship in Palliative Medicine." Journal of Palliative Medicine 10, no. 4 (2007): 938–47.

Swetz, Keith M., Sarah E. Harrington, Robin K. Matsuyama, Tait D. Shanafelt, and Laurie J. Lyckholm. "Strategies for Avoiding Burnout in Hospice and Palliative Medicine: Peer Advice for Physicians on Achieving Longevity and Fulfillment." Journal of Palliative Medicine 12, no. 9 (2009): 773–77.

Teno, Joan M., Vincent Mor, Nicholas Ward, Jason Roy, Brian Clarridge, John E. Wennberg, and Elliott S. Fisher. "Bereaved Family Member Perceptions of Quality of End-of-Life Care in U.S. Regions with High and Low Usage of Intensive Care Unit Care." Journal of the American Geriatrics Society 53, no. 11 (2005): 1905–11.

*Section 4: Decision-Making Concerning Specific Treatments and Technologies*

**Forgoing life-sustaining treatments: Ethical and practical considerations**

Arnold, Robert M. "Fast Facts and Concepts: Discussing Organ Donation with Families." Journal of Palliative Medicine 8, no. 3 (2005): 639–41.

Derse, Arthur R. "Limitation of Treatment at the End-of-Life: Withholding and Withdrawal." Clinical Geriatric Medicine 21 no. 1 (2005): 223–38.

Edwards, Miles J., and Susan W. Tolle. "Disconnecting a Ventilator at the Request of a Patient Who Knows He Will Then Die: The Doctor's Anguish." Annals of Internal Medicine 117 (1992): 254–57.

Gerstel, Eric, Ruth A. Engelberg, Thomas Koepsell, and J. Randall Curtis. "Duration of Withdrawal of Life Support in the Intensive Care Unit and Association with Family Satisfaction." American Journal of Respiratory Critical Care Medicine 178, no. 8 (2008): 798–804.

Rubenfeld, Gordon D., and J. Randall Curtis. "Improving Care for Patients Dying in the Intensive Care Unit." Clinics in Chest Medicine 24, no. 4 (2003): 763–73.

Truog, Robert D. "Consent for Organ Donation: Balancing Conflicting Ethical Obligations." NEJM 358, no. 12 (2008): 1209–11.

Truog, Robert D., Margaret L. Campbell, J. Randall Curtis, Curtis E. Haas, John M. Luce, Gordon D. Rubenfeld, Cynda H. Rushton, and David C. Kaufman. "Recommendations for End-of-Life Care in the Intensive Care Unit: A Consensus Statement by the American Academy of Critical Care Medicine." Critical Care Medicine 36, no. 3 (2008): 953–63.

Williams, Michael A., Pamela A. Lipsett, Cynda H. Rushton, Eugene C. Grochowski, Ivor D. Berkowitz, Stephen L. Mann, John H. Shatzer, Priscilla M. Short, and Myron Genel. "The Physician's Role in Discussing Organ Donation with Families." Critical Care Medicine 31, no. 5 (2003): 1568–73.

**Brain injuries and neurological states**

Bernat, James L. "Chronic Consciousness Disorders." Annual Review of Medicine 60, no. 1 (2009): 381–92.

———. *Ethical Issues in Neurology*. 3d ed. Philadelphia, PA: Lippincott, Williams and Wilkins, 2008.

———. "Ethical Issues in the Treatment of Severe Brain Injury: The Impact of New Technologies." Annals of the New York Academy of Sciences 1157 (2009): 117–30.

Cochrane, Thomas I. "Unnecessary Time Pressure in Refusal of Life-Sustaining Therapies: Fear of Missing the Opportunity to Die." American Journal of Bioethics 9, no. 4 (2009): 47–54.

Corrigan, John D., Jennifer A. Bogner, Jerry W. Mysiw, Daniel Clinchot, and Lisa Fugate. "Life Satisfaction after Traumatic Brain Injury." Journal of Head Trauma Rehabilitation 16, no. 6 (2001): 543–55.

Estraneo, Anna, Pasquale Moretta, Vincenzo Loreto, Bernardo Lanzillo, Lucio Santoro, and Luigi Trojano. "Late Recovery after Traumatic, Anoxic, or Hemorrhagic Long-Lasting Vegetative State." Neurology 75, no. 3 (2010): 239–45.

Fins, Joseph J., "Brain Injury: The Vegetative and Minimally Conscious States," in *From Birth to Death and Bench to Clinic: The Hastings Center Bioethics Briefing Book for Journalists, Policymakers, and Campaigns* (Garrison, NY: The Hastings Center, 2008).

———. "Ethics of Clinical Decision Making and Communication with Surrogates." In: *Plum and Posner's Diagnosis of Stupor and Coma*, 4th ed., ed. Jerome Posner, Clifford B. Saper, Nicholas Schiff, and Fred Plum. New York: Oxford University Press, 2007.

———. "Rethinking Disorders of Consciousness: New Research and Its Implications." Hastings Center Report 35, no. 2 (2005): 22–24.

———, Maria G. Master, Linda M. Gerber, and Joseph T. Giacino. "The Minimally Conscious State: A Diagnosis in Search of an Epidemiology." Archives of Neurology 64, no. 10 (2012): 1400–1405.

Giacino, Joseph T., Stephen Ashwal, and Nancy Childs, "The Minimally Conscious State: Definition and Diagnostic Criteria," *Neurology* 58, no. 3 (2002): 349–53.

Gill, Carol J. "Depolarizing and Complicating the Ethics of Treatment Decision Making in Brain Injury: A Disability Rights Response to Nelson and Frader." Journal of Clinical Ethics 15, no. 4 (2004): 277–88.

Jennett, Bryan. *The Vegetative State*. New York: Cambridge University Press, 2002.

———, and Fred Plum. "Persistent Vegetative State after Brain Damage. A Syndrome in Search of a Name." Lancet 299, no. 7753 (1972): 734–37.

Katz, Douglas I., Meg Polyak, Daniel Coughlan, Meliné Nichols, and Alexis Roche. "Natural History of Recovery from Brain Injury after Prolonged Disorders of Consciousness: Outcome of Patients Admitted to Inpatient Rehabilitation with 1–4 Year Follow-Up." Progress in Brain Research 177 (2009): 73–88.

Lammi, Michele H., Vanessa H. Smith, Robyn L. Tate, and Christine M. Taylor. "The Minimally Conscious State and Recovery Potential: A Follow-Up Study 2 to 5 Years after Traumatic Brain Injury." Archives of Physical Medicine and Rehabilitation 86, no. 4 (2005): 746–54.

Nelson, James Lindemann, and Joel Frader. "Brain Trauma and Surrogate Decision Making: Dogmas, Challenges, and Response." Journal of Clinical Ethics 15, no. 4 (2004): 264–76.

Pearlman, Robert A., Kevin C. Cain, Donald L. Patrick, Malka Appelbaum-Maizel, Helene E. Starks, Nancy S. Jecker, and Richard F. Uhlmann. "Insights Pertaining to Patient Assessments of States Worse than Death." Journal of Clinical Ethics 4, no. 1 (1993): 33–41.

Wilkinson, Dominic. "The Window of Opportunity: Decision Theory and the Timing of Prognostic Tests for Newborn Infants." Bioethics 23, no. 9 (2009): 503–14.

Wilson, F. Colin, J. Harpur, Tina Watson, and J.I. Morrow. "Vegetative State and Minimally Responsive Patients: Regional Survey, Long-Term Case Outcomes and Service Recommendations." NeuroRehabilitation 17, no. 3 (2002): 231–36.


**Mechanical ventilation**

American Thoracic Society. "Consensus Statement on the Respiratory Care of the Patient with Duchenne Muscular Dystrophy." American Journal of Respiratory and Critical Care Medicine 170 (2004): 456–65.

Cooke, Colin R., David L. Hotchkin, Ruth A. Engelberg, Lewis J. Rubinson, and J. Randall Curtis. "Predictors of Time to Death after Terminal Withdrawal of Mechanical Ventilation in the ICU." Chest 138, no. 2 (2010): 289–97.

Curtis, J. Randall, Deborah J. Cook, Tasnim Sinuff, Douglas B. White, Nicholas Hill, Sean P. Keenan, Joshua O. Benditt, Robert Kacmarek, Karin T. Kirchhoff, and Mitchell M. Levy. "Noninvasive Positive Pressure Ventilation in Critical and Palliative Care Settings: Understanding the Goals of Therapy." Critical Care Medicine 35, no. 3 (2007): 932–39.

Curtis, J. Randall, and Gordon D. Rubenfeld. "Improving Palliative Care for Patients in the Intensive Care Unit." Journal of Palliative Medicine 8, no. 4 (2005): 840–54.

Glavan, Bradford J., Ruth A. Engelberg, Lois Downey, and J. Randall Curtis. "Using the Medical Record to Evaluate the Quality of End-of-Life Care in the Intensive Care Unit." Critical Care Medicine 36, no. 4 (2008): 1138–46.

Isaac, Margaret, and J. Randall Curtis. "Improving Quality of Life for Patients with Terminal Respiratory Disease." Expert Review of Respiratory Medicine 3, no. 6 (2009): 597–605.

Lemoignan, Josée, and Carolyn Ells. "Amyotrophic Lateral Sclerosis and Assisted Ventilation: How Patients Decide." Palliative and Supportive Care 8 no. 2 (2010): 207–213.

Sinuff, Tasnim, Deborah J. Cook, Sean P. Keenan, Karen E. Burns, Neill K.J. Adhikari, Graeme M. Rocker, Sangeeta Mehta, Robert Kacmarek, Eva K. Kevin, and Nicholas S. Hill. "Noninvasive Ventilation for Acute Respiratory Failure Near the End of Life." Critical Care Medicine 36, no. 3 (2008): 789–94.


**Cardiopulmonary resuscitation and cardiac treatments**
*CPR*

American Society of Anesthesiologists. "Ethical Guidelines for the Anesthesia Care of Patients with Do-Not-Resuscitate Orders or Other Directives That Limit Treatment." Approved 2001, affirmed 2008. Available at: http://www.asahq.org.

Blinderman, Craig D., Eric L. Krakauer, and Mildred Z. Solomon. "Time to Revise the Approach to Determining Cardiopulmonary Resuscitation Status." JAMA 37, no. 9 (2012): 917–18.

Kazaure, Hadiza, Sanziana Roman, and Julie A. Sosa. "High Mortality in Surgical Patients with Do-Not-Resuscitate Orders." Archives of Surgery 146, no. 8 (2011): 922–28.

McIntyre, Kevin M. "Cardiopulmonary Resuscitation in Chronically Ill Patients in the Intensive Care Unit: Does Poor Outcome Justify Withholding Cardiopulmonary Resuscitation from This Group?" Archives of Internal Medicine 152, no. 11 (1992): 2181–83.

Sanders, Alan, Melissa Schepp, and Marianne Baird. "Partial Do-Not-Resuscitate Orders: A Hazard to Patient Safety and Clinical Outcomes?" Critical Care Medicine 39, no. 1 (2011): 14–18.

Tian, Jianmin, David A. Kaufman, Stuart Zarich, Paul S. Chan, Philip Ong, Yaw Amoateng-Adjepong, and Constantine A. Manthous. "Outcomes of Critically Ill Patients Who Received Cardiopulmonary Resuscitation." American Journal of Respiratory and Critical Care Medicine 182, no. 4 (2010): 501–6.

*Cardiac treatments*

Goldstein, Nathan E., Rachel Lampert, Elizabeth Bradley, Joanne Lynn, and Harlan M. Krumholz. "Management of Implantable Cardioverter Defibrillators in End-of-Life Care." Annals of Internal Medicine 141, no. 11 (2004): 835–38.

Goldstein, Nathan E., Davendra Mehta, Saima Siddiqui, Ezra Teitelbaum, Jessica Zeidman, Magdelena Singson, Elena Pe, Elizabeth H. Bradley, and R. Sean Morrison. "'That's Like an Act of Suicide': Patients' Attitudes Toward Deactivation of Implantable Defibrillators." Journal of General Internal Medicine 23, suppl. 1 (2008): 7–12.

Goldstein, Nathan E., Davendra Mehta, Ezra Teitelbaum, Elizabeth H. Bradley, and R. Sean Morrison. "'It's Like Crossing a Bridge': Complexities Preventing Physicians from Discussing Deactivation of Implantable Defibrillators at the End of Life." Journal of General Internal Medicine 23, suppl. 1 (2008): 2–6.

Goodlin, Sarah J., Timothy E. Quill, and Robert M. Arnold. "Communication and Decision-Making about Prognosis in Heart Failure Care." Journal of Cardiac Failure 14, no. 2 (2008): 106–13.

Lampert, Rachel, David L. Hayes, George J. Annas, Margaret A. Farley, Nathan E. Goldstein, Robert M. Hamilton, G. Neal Kay, Daniel B. Kramer, Paul S. Mueller, Luigi Padeletti, Leo Pozuelo, Mark H. Schoenfeld, Panos E. Vardas, Debra L. Wiegand, and Richard Zellner. "HRS Expert Consensus Statement on the Management of Cardiovascular Implantable Electronic Devices (CIEDs) in Patients Nearing End of Life or Requesting Withdrawal of Therapy." Heart Rhythm 7, no. 7 (2010): 1008–26.

Lewis, Williams R., Donna L. Luebke, Nancy J. Johnson, Michael D. Harrington, Ottorino Costantini, and Mark P. Aulisio. "Withdrawing Implantable Defibrillator Shock Therapy in Terminally Ill Patients." American Journal of Medicine 119, no. 10 (2006): 892–96.

Lietz, Katherine. "Destination Therapy: Patient Selection and Current Outcomes." Journal of Cardiac Surgery 25, no. 4 (2010): 462–71.

———, and Leslie W. Miller. "Patient Selection for Left-Ventricular Assist Devices." Current Opinion in Cardiology 24, no. 3 (2009): 246–51.

Mueller, Paul S., Keith M. Swetz, Monica R. Freeman, Kari A. Carter, Mary E. Crowley, Cathy J. Anderson Severson, Soon J. Park, and Daniel P. Sulmasy. "Ethical Analysis of Withdrawing Ventricular Assist Device Support." Mayo Clinic Proceedings 85, no. 9 (2010): 791–97.

Sherazi, Saadia, James P. Daubert, Robert C. Block, Vinodh Jeevanantham, Khalid Abdel-Gadir, Michael R. DiSalle, James M. Haley, and Abrar H. Shah. "Physicians' Preferences and Attitudes about End-of-Life Care in Patients with an Implantable Cardioverter-Difibrillator." Mayo Clinic Proceedings 83, no. 10 (2008): 1139–41.

Sulmasy, Daniel P. "Within You/Without You: Biotechnology, Ontology, and Ethics." Journal of General Internal Medicine 23, suppl. 1 (2008): 69–72.

**Dialysis**

Cohen, Lewis M., Michael J. Germain, and David M. Poppel. "Practical Considerations in Dialysis Withdrawal: 'To Have That Option Is a Blessing.'" JAMA 289, no. 16 (2003): 2113–19.

Holley, Jean L., Sara N. Davison, and Alvin H. Moss. "Nephrologists' Changing Practices in Reported End-of-Life Decision-Making." Clinical Journal of the American Society of Nephrology 2, no. 1 (2007): 107–11.

Moss, Alvin H. "Revised Dialysis Clinical Practice Guideline Promotes More Informed Decision-Making." Clinical Journal of the American Society of Nephrology 5, no. 12 (2010): 2380–83.

———. "Shared Decision Making in Dialysis: A New Clinical Practice Guideline to Assist with Dialysis-Related Ethics Consultations." Journal of Clinical Ethics 12, no. 4 (2001): 406–14.

Murtagh, Fliss, Lewis M. Cohen, and Michael J. Germain. "Dialysis Discontinuation: Quo Vadis?" Advances in Chronic Kidney Diseases 14, no. 4 (2007): 379–401.

Renal Physician Association. *Shared Decision-Making in the Appropriate Initiation and Withdrawal from Dialysis Clinical Practice Guidelines.* 2d ed. Rockville, MD: Renal Physician Association, 2010.

Schell, Jane O., Michael J. Germain, Fred O. Finkelstein, and Lewis M. Cohen. "An Integrative Approach to the Elderly with Advanced Kidney Disease." Advances in Chronic Kidney Diseases 17, no. 4 (2010): 368–77.

**Nutrition and hydration**

Cervo, Frank A., Leslie Bryan, and Sharon Farber, "To PEG or Not to PEG: A Review of Evidence for Placing Feeding Tubes in Advanced Dementia and the Decision-Making Process." Geriatrics 61, no. 6 (2006): 30–35.

Diekema, Douglas S., Jeffrey R. Botkin, and the American Academy of Pediatrics Committee on Bioethics. "Forgoing Medically Provided Nutrition and Hydration in Children." Pediatrics 124, no. 2 (2009): 813–22.

Finucane, Thomas E., Colleen Christmas, and Kathy Travis. "Tube Feeding in Patients with Advanced Dementia: A Review of the Evidence." JAMA 282, no. 14 (1999): 1365–70.

Ganzini, Linda. "Artificial Nutrition and Hydration at the End of Life: Ethics and Evidence." Palliative and Supportive Care 4 ( 2006): 135–43.

Gillick, Muriel R. "The Use of Advance Care Planning to Guide Decisions about Artificial Nutrition and Hydration." Nutrition in Clinical Practice 21, no. 2 (2006): 126–33.

———, and Angelo E. Volandes. "The Standard of Caring: Why Do We Still Use Feeding Tubes in Patients with Advanced Dementia?" Journal of the American Medical Directors Association 9, no. 5 (2008): 364–67.

Palecek, Eric J., Joan M. Teno, David J. Casarett, Laura C. Hanson, Ramona L. Rhodes, and Susan L. Mitchell. "Comfort Feeding Only: A Proposal to Bring Clarity to Decision-Making Regarding Difficulty with Eating for Persons with Advanced Dementia." Journal of the American Geriatrics Society 58, no. 3 (2010): 580–84.

### Chemotherapy and other cancer treatments

Brumley, Richard, Susan Enguidanos, Paula Jamison, Rae Seitz, Nora Morgenstern, Sherry Saito, Jan McIlwane, Kristine Hillary, and Jorge Gonzalez. "Increased Satisfaction with Care and Lower Costs: Results of a Randomized Trial of In-Home Palliative Care." Journal of the American Geriatrics Society 55, no. 7 (2007): 993–1000.

Connor, Stephen R., Bruce Pyenson, Kathryn Fitch, Carol Spence, and Kosuke Iwasaki. "Comparing Hospice and Nonhospice Patient Survival among Patients Who Die within a Three-Year Window." Journal of Pain and Symptom Management 33, no. 3 (2007): 238–46.

Gade, Glenn, Ingrid Venohr, Douglas Conner, Kathleen McGrady, Jeffrey Beane, Robert H. Richardson, Marilyn P. Williams, Marcia Liberson, Mark Blum, and Richard Della Penna. "Impact of an Inpatient Palliative Care Team: A Randomized Control Trial." Journal of Palliative Medicine 11, no. 2 (2008): 180–90.

Gawande, Atul. "Letting Go: What Should Medicine Do When It Can't Save Your Life?" New Yorker 86, no. 22 (2010): 36–49.

Harrington, Sarah E., and Thomas J. Smith. "The Role of Chemotherapy at the End of Life: 'When Is Enough, Enough?'" JAMA 99, no. 22 (2008): 2667–78.

Keating, Nancy L., Mary Beth Landrum, Selwyn O. Rogers, Susan K. Baum, Beth A. Virnig, Haiden A. Huskamp, Craig C. Earle, and Katherine L. Kahn. "Physician Factors Associated with Discussions about End-of-Life Care." Cancer 116, no. 4 (2010): 998–1006.

Matsuyama, Robin, Sashidhar Reddy, and Thomas J. Smith. "Why Do Patients Choose Chemotherapy Near the End of Life? A Review of the Perspective of Those Facing Death from Cancer." Journal of Clinical Oncology 24, no. 21 (2006): 3490–96.

Peppercorn, Jeffrey M., Thomas J. Smith, Paul R. Helft, David J. Debono, Scott R. Berry, Dana S. Wollins, Daniel M. Hayes, Jamie H. Von Roenn, and Lowell E. Schnipper. "American Society of Clinical Oncology Statement: Toward Individualized Care for Patients with Advanced Cancer." Journal of Clinical Oncology 29, no. 6 (2011): 755–60.

Reisfield, Gary M., and George R. Wilson. "Use of Metaphor in the Discourse on Cancer." Journal of Clinical Oncology 22, no. 19 (2004): 4024–27.

Smith, Thomas J., Sarah Temin, Erin R. Alesi, Amy P. Abernethy, Tracy A. Balboni, Ethan M. Basch, Betty R. Ferrell, Matt Loscalzo, Diane E. Meier, Judith A. Paice, Jeffery M. Peppercorn, Mark Somerfield, Ellen Stovall, and Jamie H. Von Roenn. "American Society of Clinical Oncology Provisional Clinical Opinion: The Integration of Palliative Care into Standard Oncology Care." Journal of Clinical Oncology 30, no. 8 (2012): 880–87.

Weeks, Jane C., Paul J. Catalano, Angel Cronin, Matthew D. Finkelman, Jennifer W. Mack, Nancy L. Keating, and Deborah Schrag. "Patients' Expectations about Effects of Chemotherapy for Advanced Cancer." NEJM 367, no. 17 (2012): 1616–25. See also: Smith, Thomas J. and Dan L. Longo. "Talking with Patients about Dying." NEJM 367, no. 17 (2012): 1651–52.

### Routine medications, antibiotics, and invasive procedures

Currow, David C., James P. Stevenson, Amy P. Abernethy, John Plummer, and Tania M. Shelby-James. "Prescribing in Palliative Care as Death Approaches." Journal of the American Geriatrics Society 55, no. 4 (2007): 590–95.

Givens, Jane L., Rich N. Jones, Michele L. Shaffer, Dan K. Kiely, and Susan L. Mitchell. "Survival and Comfort after Treatment of Pneumonia in Advanced Dementia." Archives of Internal Medicine 170, no. 13 (2010): 1102–7.

Hill, Robin R., Kerri D. Martinez, Thomas Delate, and Daniel M. Witt. "A Descriptive Evaluation of Warfarin Use in Patients Receiving Hospice or Palliative Care Services." Journal of Thrombosis and Thrombolysis 27, no. 3 (2009): 334–39.

Holmes, Holly M., Kevin T. Bain, Ali Zalpour, Ruili Luo, Eduardo Bruera, and James S. Goodwin. "Predictors of Anticoagulation in Hospice Patients with Lung Cancer." Cancer 116, no. 20 (2010): 4817–24.

Smith, Alexander K., Mara A. Schonberg, Jonathan Fisher, Daniel J. Pallin, Susan D. Block, Lachlan Forrow, and Ellen P. McCarthy. "Emergency Department Experiences of Acutely Symptomatic Patients with Terminal Illness and Their Family Caregivers." Journal of Pain and Symptom Management 39, no. 6 (2010): 972–81.

Spiess, Jeffrey L. "Can I Stop the Warfarin? A Review of the Risk and Benefits of Discontinuing Anticoagulation." Journal of Palliative Medicine 12, no. 1 (2009): 83–87.

Tjia, Jennifer, Margaret R. Rothman, Dan K. Kiely, Michele L. Shaffer, Holly M. Holmes, Greg A. Sachs, and Susan L. Mitchell. "Daily Medication Use in Nursing Home Residents with Advanced Dementia." Journal of the American Geriatrics Society 58, no. 5 (2010): 880–88.

Vollrath, Annette M., Christian Sinclair, and James Hallenbeck. "Discontinuing Cardiovascular Medications at the End of Life: Lipid-Lowering Agents." Journal of Palliative Medicine 8, no. 4 (2005): 876–81.

**Blood transfusion and blood products**

Doyle, John D. "Blood Transfusions and the Jehovah's Witness Patient." American Journal of Therapeutics 9, no. 5 (2002): 417–24.

Hughes, Duncan B., Brant W. Ullery, and Philip S. Barie. "The Contemporary Approach to the Care of Jehovah's Witnesses." Journal of Trauma 65, no. 1 (2008): 237–47.

Knuti, Kristine A., Philip C. Amrein, Bruce A. Chabner, Thomas J. Lynch, Jr., and Richard T. Penson. "Faith, Identity, and Leukemia: When Blood Products Are Not an Option." Oncologist 7, no. 4 (2002): 371–80.

Rogers, David M., and Kendall P. Crookston. "The Approach to the Patient Who Refuses Blood Transfusion." Transfusion 46, no. 9 (2006): 1471–77.

**Palliative sedation**

Boyle, Joseph. "Medical Ethics and Double Effect: The Case of Terminal Sedation." Theoretical Medicine and Bioethics 25, no. 1 (2004): 51–60.

Carr, Mark F., and Gina Jervey Mohr. "Palliative Sedation as Part of the Continuum of Palliative Care." Journal of Palliative Medicine 11, no. 1 (2008): 76–81.

Carver, Alan C., and Kathleen M. Foley. "Symptom Assessment and Management." Neurologic Clinics 19, no. 4 (2001): 921–47.

Cherny, Nathan L., and Russell K. Portenoy. "Sedation in the Management of Refractory Symptoms: Guidelines for Evaluation and Treatment." Journal of Palliative Care 10, no. 2 (1994): 31–38.

Jansen, Lynn A., and Daniel P. Sulmasy. "Sedation, Hydration, Alimentation, and Equivocation: Careful Conversation about Care at the End of Life." Annals of Internal Medicine 136, no. 11 (2002): 845–49.

Kirk, Timothy W., and Margaret M. Mahon. "National Hospice and Palliative Care Organization (NHPCO) Position Statement and Commentary on the Use of Palliative Sedation in Imminently Dying Terminally Ill Patients." Journal of Pain and Symptom Management 39, no. 5 (2010): 914–23.

Levy, Michael H., and Seth D. Cohen. "Sedation for the Relief of Refractory Symptoms in the Imminently Dying: A Fine Intentional Line." Seminars in Oncology 32, no. 2 (2005): 237–46.

Lo, Bernard, and Gordon Rubenfeld. "Palliative Sedation in Dying Patients: 'We Turn to It When Everything Else Hasn't Worked.'" JAMA 294, no. 14 (2005): 1810–16.

National Ethics Committee, Veterans Health Administration. "The Ethics of Palliative Sedation as a Therapy of Last Resort." American Journal of Hospice and Palliative Care 23, no. 6 (2007): 483–91.

Quill, Timothy E., and Ira R. Byock. "Responding to Intractable Terminal Suffering: The Role of Terminal Sedation and Voluntary Refusal of Food and Fluids." Annals of Internal Medicine 132, no. 5 (2000): 408–14. See also: Yannow, Morton Leonard. "Responding to Intractable Suffering." Annals of Internal

Medicine 132, no. 7 (2000): 560; Krakauer, Eric. "Responding to Intractable Suffering." Annals of Internal Medicine 133, no. 7 (2000): 560; Sulmasy, Daniel P., Wayne A. Ury, Judith C. Ahronheim, Mark Siegler, Leon Kass, John Lantos, Robert A. Burt, Kathleen Foley, Richard Payne, Carlos Gomez, Thomas J. Krizek, Edmund D. Pellegrino, and Russell K. Portenoy. "Responding to Intractable Suffering." Annals of Internal Medicine 133, no. 7 (2000): 560–61; and Quill, Timothy E., and Ira R. Byock. "Responding to Intractable Suffering." Annals of Internal Medicine 133, no. 7 (2000): 561–62.

*Section 5: Institutional Discussion Guide on Resource Allocation and the Cost of Care*

Council on Ethical and Judicial Affairs, American Medical Association. "Ethical Issues in Health Care Systems Reform: The Provision of Adequate Health Care." JAMA 272, no. 13 (1994): 1056–62.

Daniels, Norman, and James E. Sabin. *Setting Limits Fairly: Learning to Share Resources for Health*. New York: Oxford University Press, 2008.

Fojo, Tito, and Christine Grady. "How Much Is Life Worth: Cetuximab, Non-Small Cell Lung Cancer, and the $440 Billion Question." Journal of the National Cancer Institute 101, no. 15 (2009): 1044–48.

Gilmer, Todd, Lawrence J. Schneiderman, Holly Teetzel, Jeffrey Blustein, Kathleen Briggs, Felicia Cohn, Ronald Cranford, Daniel Dugan, Glen Komatsu, and Ernlé Young. "The Costs of Non-Beneficial Treatment in the Intensive Care Setting." Health Affairs 24, no. 4 (2005): 961–71.

Goodman, David C., Elliott S. Fisher, Chiang-Hua Chang, Nancy E. Morden, Joseph O. Jacobson, Kimberly Murray, and Susan Miesfeldt. *Quality of End-of-Life Cancer Care for Medicare Beneficiaries: Regional and Hospital-Specific Analysis*. Hanover, NH: The Dartmouth Institute for Health Policy and Clinical Practice, 2010.

Hillner, Bruce E., and Thomas J Smith. "Efficacy Does Not Necessarily Translate to Cost Effectiveness: A Case Study in the Challenges Associated with 21st-Century Cancer Drug Pricing." Journal of Clinical Oncology 27, no. 13 (2009): 2111–13.

Hogan, Christopher, June Lunney, Jon Gabel, and Joanne Lynn. "Medicare Beneficiaries' Costs of Care in the Last Year of Life." Health Affairs 20, no. 4 (2001): 188–95.

Jennings, Bruce, and Mary Beth Morrissey. "Health Care Costs in End-of-Life and Palliative Care: The Quest for Ethical Reform." Journal of Social Work in End-Of-Life & Palliative Care 7, no. 4 (2011): 300–317.

Mechanic, David. "Muddling Through Elegantly: Finding the Proper Balance in Rationing." Health Affairs 16, no. 5 (1997): 83–92.

Neumann, Peter J., Jennifer A. Palmer, Eric Nadler, Chihui Fang, and Peter Ubel. "Cancer Therapy Costs Influence Treatment: A National Survey of Oncologists." Health Affairs 29, no. 1 (2010): 196–202.

Persad, Govind, Alan Wertheimer, and Ezekiel J. Emanuel. "Principles for Allocation of Scarce Medical Interventions." Lancet 373, no. 9661 (2009): 423–31.

Sulmasy, Daniel P. "Physicians, Cost Control, and Ethics." Annals of Internal Medicine 116, no. 11 (1992): 920–26.

Tangka, Florence K., Justin G. Trogdon, Lisa C. Richardson, David Howard, Susan A. Sabatino, and Eric A. Finkelstein. "Cancer Treatment Cost in the United States: Has the Burden Shifted Over Time?" Cancer 116, no. 14 (2010): 3477–84.

Ubel, Peter A., and Susan Goold. "Recognizing Bedside Rationing: Clear Cases and Tough Calls." Annals of Internal Medicine 126, no. 1 (1997): 74–80.

Zhang, Baohui, Alexi A. Wright, Haiden A. Huskamp, Matthew E. Nilsson, Matthew L. Maciejewski, Craig C. Earle, Susan D. Block, Paul K. Maciejewski, and Holly G. Prigerson. "Health Care Costs in the Last Week of Life: Associations with End-of-Life Conversations." Archives of Internal Medicine 169, no. 5 (2009): 480–88.

**Undocumented immigrants and access to life-sustaining treatment**

Campbell, G. Adam, Scott Sanoff, and Mitchell H. Rosner. "Care of the Undocumented Immigrant in the United States with ESRD." American Journal of Kidney Diseases 55, no. 1 (2009): 181–91.

Coritsidis, George N., Hasan Khamash, Shaheena I. Ahmed, Abdel-Moneim Attia, Pedro Rodriguez, Melitza K. Kiroycheva, and Nahid Ansari. "The Initiation of Dialysis in Undocumented Aliens: The Impact on a Public Hospital System." American Journal of Kidney Diseases 43, no. 3 (2004): 424–32.

Coyle, Susan. "Providing Care to Undocumented Immigrants." The Hospitalist (July–August 2003): 24–27.

Hurley, Laura, Allison Kempe, Lori A. Crane, Arthur Davidson, Katherine Pratte, Stuart Linas, L. Miriam Dickinson, and Tomas Berl. "Care of Undocumented Individuals with ESRD: A National Survey of U.S. Nephrologists." American Journal of Kidney Diseases 53, no. 6 (2009): 940–49.

Nuila, Ricardo. "Home: Palliation for Dying Undocumented Immigrants." NEJM 366, no. 22 (2012): 2047–48.

Raghavan, Rajeev, and Ricardo Nuila. "Survivors—Dialysis, Immigration, and U.S. Law." NEJM 364, no. 23 (2011): 2183–85.

Zuckerman, Stephen, Timothy A. Waidmann, and Emily Lawton. "Undocumented Immigrants, Left Out of Health Reform, Likely to Continue to Grow as Share of the Uninsured." Health Affairs 30, no. 10 (2011): 197–204.

# Index